Journey

to

WHOLENESS

And the day came when the risk to remain tight in a bud
was more painful than the risk it took to bloom.

by

Barbara Marie Brewster

FOUR WINDS PUBLISHING

ACKNOWLEDGMENTS

Although everything in this book is true, some names have been changed in order to honor the privacy of those concerned.

Cover Quote: Author Unknown

Cover Design: Therese Heyndrickx, Karen Downs, Richard Ferguson.

Rose Designs: Therese Heyndrickx

Publication Information for sources of quotes used in the text is contained in the reading list.

ISBN: O-96286O8-1-6

Publisher's Cataloging in Publication
(Prepared by Quality Books Inc.)

Brewster, Barbara M.
Journey to wholeness : and the day came when the risk to remain tight in a bud was more painful than the risk it took to bloom / Barbara Marie Brewster.
p. cm.
Includes bibliographical references.
ISBN O-96286O8-1-6

1. Self-help techniques--Biography. 2. Autobiography--Women authors. 3. Psychotherapy. I. Title.

BF632 158.1 QBI91-1541

Published by
FOUR WINDS PUBLICATIONS
6267 S.W. Miles Ct., Portland, OR, 97219
Phone: (503) 246-9424. FAX: (503) 246-9497

WHAT PEOPLE SAY ABOUT *JOURNEY TO WHOLENESS*

This book is dynamite. It just exploded for me. It's the best self-help book I've ever read. It deals with many of the things I'm going through right now. I know that reading ***Journey to Wholeness*** will change people's lives. It is THE resource book--I want to buy a case of them to give to everyone I know.

Eileen Whitelaw, counselor and administrator.

A touching, deeply intimate account. This book should not be missed by anyone interested in the journey toward health and wholeness.

Larry Krantz, M.D., director, Whole Health Institute, Colorado.

Journey to Wholeness is an incredible adventure of healing and transformation. Barbara Brewster writes from the heart and speaks with the authority only acquired by one who is living life fully. As a person who understands universal truth, she is now "passing it on" so others might learn from her experience.

Reverend Mary Manin Boggs, director, Living Enrichment Center, Portland, Oregon

I, too, have habits, patterns and behaviors that don't serve me and that I want to change. ***Journey to Wholeness*** tells me that I can do that.

A 63-year-old woman.

An honest, moving chronicle of how meaning enters illness and why healing, if complete, must address life's meanings. ***Journey to Wholeness*** will encourage and enlighten anyone interested in true healing.

Larry Dossey, M.D., author of Meaning and Medicine, Recovering the Soul, and Beyond Illness.

A courageous woman's transformation unfolds as she endeavors to discover the relationships of mind, body, emotion and spirit to a disease that threatens to overtake her life. These become revealed as she tells her story with profound clarity.

Joy Young, Ph.D.

Ever since I read ***Journey to Wholeness***, I've been thinking and thinking about what it said. It's encouraged me to do some things that are important for me--and I've decided to go back to school and get my masters degree in marketing and sales--which I love.

A new mother.

What a delight it is to read this new and important contribution to the field of healing. The path Barbara Brewster followed is practically identical to my own concept of a therapy of the Whole Person developed in the course of over 30 years' experience at Meadowlark.

In dealing with a chronic illness commonly accepted by the medical profession as being incurable, Barbara Brewster has led the reader along her own path to recovery. She has demonstrated the great power of love in the field of healing. In respect to the body, this meant proper nutrition; in the case of the mind, there was needed cleansing of the pollution from retained memories of guilt, unforgiveness and stored up anger. This was followed by the visualization of her own new body-mind image along with the courage to accept herself as she was, on a new unique path toward the liberation of her True Self.

Evarts Loomis, M.D., founder of Meadowlark holistic retreat center, California.

I read ***Journey to Wholeness*** with deep appreciation. It's probably the most honest book ever written.

Frances Horn, Ph.D., author of "I Want One Thing."

Journey to Wholeness changed my life ... I've read it three times now. I keep reading it because Barbara Brewster's example tells me that I, too, can heal.

A woman who has undergone terrible body changes similar to the symptoms of MS.

CONTENTS

DEDICATION

It was a delightfully hot August day. Sweat mixed with dirt and ran down my face. Mud and bark dust smudged my shorts and strong, tan legs. For a final time I maneuvered the wheelbarrow into position and swiftly hefted the last of the new fir trees into the hole I had just dug. Suddenly the phone rang. Putting down my shovel, I picked up the outside phone and sat on the patio chair.

Katherine, one of my dearest friends, was calling from Australia. Her voice sounded unnaturally high-pitched as she explained, "Barbara, my niece in Germany has MS ... She just found out ... She's only 26 and totally shattered by this devastating news ... Would you write to her about your experience with MS? .... Your example will encourage her that she, too, can beat this thing ... Please help her."

After we had talked for nearly an hour, I put down the phone and sat quietly in the afternoon sun. How could I be of help from 10,000 miles away? I began to recall the shattering days when my body first crashed and my world turned upside down. Looking at the dirt under my fingernails, I was struck, as I always am, by the miracle of today's healthy body--a strong body that savors heady, sweaty racquetball games and high mountain hikes, an energetic body that thinks nothing of plunging into strenuous yard work and then pausing to swim a mile. It's also a cooperative body, supporting me in labors I love, carrying me into circumstances of heartful sharing with special people, and bearing me on adventures that extend to the ends of the earth. This body of today, which I nurture, appreciate and celebrate, is an incredible contrast to the weak, confused and disintegrating body which I believed had betrayed me and which I once hated.

Images of the last six years whirled through my mind ... of doctors, workshops, books, counselors, therapies, all the desperate efforts to get well. Out of the images there emerged a clear picture of how I could help Katherine's niece. I knew that sharing the experience of my journey from that difficult place to the wondrous wholeness of today would be the most valuable and loving gift I could offer.

My purpose in sharing my journey, first with Katherine's niece and now with you, is not to extol the difficulties of a particular health problem. Rather, it is to remind and affirm, for myself and for all who are undergoing difficulties, that we can look beyond labels and the fears which they invoke, and recognize that vast choices exist. We each have infinite options for how we conduct the nature of the journey. I believe that the choices I made and how I addressed my dis-ease have brought me to a place, not only of restored harmony, but of renewal, rebirth, re-creation.

Whether my present condition is labeled "cured" or "remission" doesn't matter to me. The truth is that today I display classic symptoms of health, energy, happiness--none of which I take for granted. I accept the responsibility which my renewed well-being lays upon me. The task of creating and maintaining wholeness of body, mind and spirit is an ever-evolving, life-long activity. In this, too, I have choices.

I dedicate this book to Katherine's niece and to you who, by accepting the challenge of your ordeal, whatever it may be, have courageously embarked upon your own unique journey to wholeness and blossoming. My desire is to urge you to look beyond the despair, to inspire you to embrace the resources around and within you, and to excite you about where you can go.

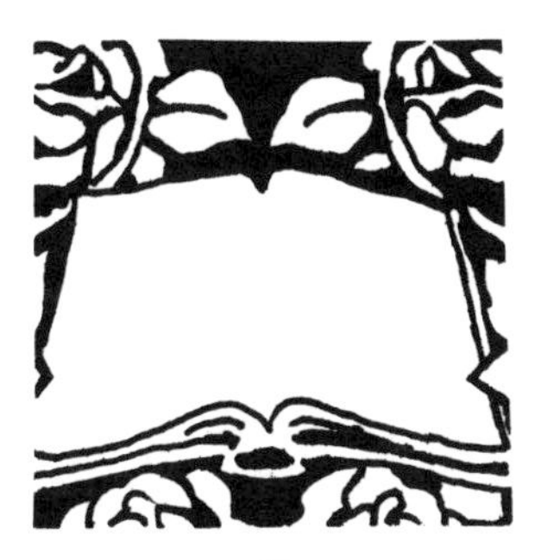

PART I

BECOMING MY OWN MENTOR

We are faced with the reality that if we wish to live fully and in harmony with life, we will have to become self-motivated students. We will have to be ready to risk, look inside ourselves, and proceed through trial and error. The job will be mainly ours. We will be required to be our own mentors.

Leo Buscaglia, ***Personhood***

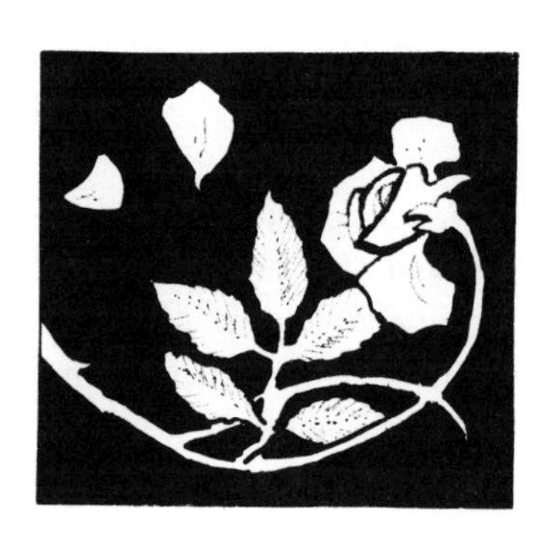

CHAPTER ONE

IN AUGUST 1983, I attended my 20 year high school reunion, a woman who had apparently settled into the fold of the American Dream. No signs remained of the wanderlust of my twenties, of the girl who emigrated to Australia and performed gymnastics in Denmark, who hitchhiked on airplanes and Mack trucks and hostessed a restaurant in Afghanistan. After 13 years of marriage to a gentle but fireless man, I owned a successful business, played A class racquetball, was progressing in singing lessons, sported a tan, tight-toned body, and had parents who occasionally helped out financially.

In the same way that soldiers remember the date that war was declared, I shall always remember the day when my life changed. On September 18 the first tingling ran down my right arm, soon to follow down my legs, down my other arm and across my face. As I tried to believe it was just a pinched nerve, perhaps from racquetball, a part of me froze inside, intuiting that my life would never be the same again. It wasn't until a year later that the bizarre and painful symptoms that plagued me were diagnosed as multiple sclerosis.

Crisis, I believe, calls for something from us--to open to whatever is necessary to restore or create harmony. In my case, what was called for was a metamorphosis. It was a process in which I underwent the very hard work of dying to the old self and replacing it with a new, untried self; a process in which I oscillated between triumphs and discouragement as I consciously broke down limiting beliefs and behaviors and risked trying fresh ones.

Although MS was the spur to my self-change, the issue was not so much about recovering from disease. It would soon become evident that the issue was more about recovering from the misbeliefs, fears, doubts and self-inflicted limitations that characterized the climate of my life.

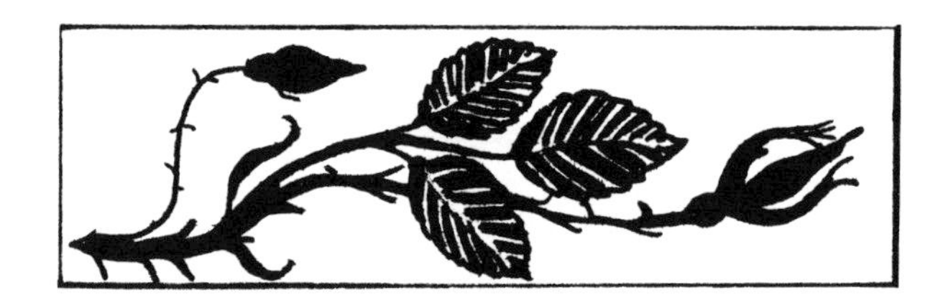

When it all started, I couldn't understand what was happening. For 38 years I had taken my health for granted. Now, all at once, my body seemed to be going completely haywire. The first indication that something was wrong appeared on the racquetball court. For no apparent reason, I was missing the overhead shots. Within the space of a few days, my accuracy and power dissipated and, seemingly overnight, I became a sloppy, weak player. Then came the tingling feelings in my arms, legs and face. By the end of September, my energy was totally depleted. My legs felt so shaky that I was surprised I didn't fall down. Burning pain raged across my back and hips. Pins and needles coursed in waves along my arms and legs. Some unseen enemy was stalking and attacking me, and I felt helpless to identify or arrest it.

I embarked on a cycle of endless rounds of doctor visits but was given no organic reasons for my distress. A rheumatologist suggested that I had fibrositis. "You fit the profile," he said, and went on to explain, "People with this condition are usually women in their thirties. They have poor sleep patterns and tend to be particularly accomplishment oriented. There is no cure. The only way to relieve it is to remove the stresses."

When I took the time--and the courage--to scrutinize myself honestly, I had to acknowledge that there were many conditions in my life that were stressful. The two biggest stresses were my marriage and my business.

Jack and I had been married for 13 years. I cared for him, but we were mismatched. I loved such pursuits as growth seminars, hitchhiking, plunging nude into mountain pools and meeting new people. Jack was comfortable with the known and the predictable. He had his racquetball club; I joined my own. While he went hunting, I went to philosophy lectures. He preferred meat and potatoes; I pursued natural foods. On the surface we were polite, but underneath a widening chasm separated us.

I was unhappy staying with Jack, but I didn't know how to leave. For several years I had wrestled with the decision of what to do. Could I leave without hurting him? How did I know this wasn't the normal course of relationships anyway? Wouldn't I be exchanging a good man for years of loneliness?

The other major stress was my dried flower shop which had become a unique, fantasy-filled, Portland landmark. Despite the shop's colorful charm and beauty, in eight years of business I was constantly working against time, unable to catch my breath, and was pushing myself to ever more commitments. Just as with the marriage, I didn't know how to extricate myself. Where would the money come from? What would I do? How could I throw away a successful enterprise, an investment of years?

Throughout 1983, Jack and I took steps to resolve our situation. We entered into many gut-wrenching conversations, saw a counselor, and tried to work together to understand our differences. It was a stressful, sad and difficult process. In April of 1984 we separated.

Because the marriage and my poor health preoccupied me so thoroughly, I couldn't begin to deal with the business problems. I muddled along, vacillating between attempts to liquidate the shop, sell it, or improve it. Although I knew it needed a resolution, the business remained.

My health did not improve and I sought answers from countless directions. From one doctor, I learned about *Candida albicans*, allergies, and how the immune system becomes depleted. I read books about candida and learned that it is a yeast which is present in everyone's body. Under certain conditions it can run rampant and over-colonize, causing multiple and varied symptoms such as those which I had.

Hand in hand with candida went allergies. To my dismay, testing revealed that many common foods and chemicals were poison to my body. I had to relearn how to eat. Foods such as wheat, yeast, sugar, dairy products, nightshades (tomatoes, potatoes, green peppers, eggplant), coffee, tea, baking powder, corn and soy were eliminated from my diet. In addition, all detergents, perfumes, soaps, cleaning agents and chemicals were removed from my house.

For the next year I exhausted myself exploring therapies--restricting my foods, forcing myself to stretch and walk when I didn't have the energy, reading endless books and articles on nutrition and preventative medicine, seeking guidance from neurologists, naturopaths, osteopaths, M.D.'s and more. Every small step forward seemed to yield two steps back. No matter how strict my diet or how much I tried to resolve my stresses, nothing seemed to change. In fact, the overall picture just got worse.

Gradually, a shift took place--a shift from looking outside myself for wellness to looking within. I had been seeking relief and solutions in externals--thinking if I could only alter *other* people, change my marriage, my business, my food, my sleeping, my bank account, my muscle tone--then I would be well. I started considering the possibility that what was happening in my life was a sign of inner disharmony--and that something more than mere physical modifications was necessary. I needed to change at other levels--to release outmoded habits, establish more wholesome behavior patterns, reorder my beliefs, turn inward, trust, and surrender to a higher power. I had no idea how to do this or where the process would take me.

> *"I would be making a journey, an essentially lonely journey, into myself, in search of something that was meaningful to me alone. In that journey my friends would be my enemies, my enjoyments would be my liabilities, and the blandishments of society in general would be impediments to any change. I had to see life differently, yet I had mixed feelings about the new path I was taking."*
>
> *David Smith,* ***Healing Journey***

CHAPTER TWO

IT WAS MAY 1984, a month after Jack and I had separated. A friend loaned me the book, *I Want One Thing*. It spoke to me as I cast about for the answers to my questions about what I should do.

The book was written by a 74-year-old woman, Frances Horn, whose desire for wholeness paralleled mine. She found that when she acted in accordance with being open to WHATEVER would be the appropriate self-fulfilling thing, then she lived positively. When she was not centered and not willing to listen to WHATEVER was appropriate, then her life was very difficult.

As I looked at the decisions before me I realized that I had to make the choice to allow WHATEVER expressed wholeness to be the ruling factor. That meant that I had to release my attachment to specific desires and to cease demanding or expecting particular outcomes. Only then would I be in a state of willingness--to accept WHATEVER the appropriate response might be moment by moment. I would then be shifting to an *inner* consciousness, to an intuitive knowing. I gave it the freedom to speak clearly to me when I only wanted "one thing"--to hear what it had to say to me, and to act accordingly.

In regard to the flower shop, I asked myself, *What is the appropriate response for me?* The answer came, *It's WHATEVER I see to do when I let go of all specifics--when I am no longer holding on to narrow attachments. It is what offers itself as an answer when I am truly open to allowing WHATEVER wants to express through me in the creative moment.* With this realization, I began to step across the threshold of learning to trust. If I was going to choose to express wholeness, then I had to trust that, somehow, something would guide me into the concrete and specific actions which would lead me there. I had to trust that each moment called for something from me, and that my openness to it would allow me to see what that was.

I read on. I skipped the newspaper. I didn't go to work. I didn't walk, so important was it for me to follow through with this concept. I applied it to my shop decision, asking myself, *Am I willing to do WHATEVER is appropriate for me at this moment?*

Yes.

What is appropriate?

What is appropriate is my self-fullfillment, and I'm not attaining that in the present situation. The appropriate thing for me is to move on, to drop the negating influences that the business has on me.

This was a huge new awareness--opening to the realization that under all the confusions and issues and questions and busyness I really only wanted "one thing"--self-fulfillment. But what *was* self-fulfillment? I couldn't begin to answer that. I only knew that, clearly, I was far from it in my present state.

Let go of my attachments to the specifics! I told myself. *To my pride, to achievement, money and recognition, to the present momentum, to my fear of what to do next. I have no idea how I will achieve self-fulfillment, but I do know that I've been at the flower shop for ten years and haven't found it.*

How little did I realize what I was committing myself to. How could I imagine the extent to which I would be forced to let go of specifics, or the degree to which I would be required to trust. How naive I was to think that this enterprise of releasing attachments and the outmoded would proceed in the breezy romantic way that I envisioned. How little I knew of the ways the world has of breaking apart and tearing away the worn foundations--or of the enormity of the task of being reestablished in an unfamiliar form. Little did I know that I was about to be thrust into the fire, melted down, emptied and purified and molded anew.

How thankful I was for the appearance of Frances Horn's book just then. Frances' experience of being open to WHATEVER helped tremendously as I learned to do the same. I began making decisions without laboring and flip-flopping. I just checked if something seemed right for the situation--and I did it. *Even if it turns out "wrong,"* I told myself, *I can be assured that I am still moving forward and am on my path. At least I will stop making my life miserable by incessantly agonizing about decisions.*

Looking for friendship on a low day, I phoned my friend, Leith, in Phoenix. Although Leith and I were the same age, Leith's flaxen hair and China blue eyes gave the impression of a beautiful porcelain doll. Her apparent wide-eyed innocence, however, belied the underlying earthiness and razor-sharp intelligence that had led her to become a bank executive, scholar, teacher and a unique mother. Now, her soft, calm voice warmly welcomed and supported me. After we had talked a while, she said, "My son, Todd, wants me to join him on a ten day Sikh Retreat in New Mexico. There will be yoga and meditation and five days of silence. Why don't you come?"

Neither Leith nor I had any idea what the Sikhs and their retreat would be like, but the idea of sunny New Mexico and of stepping out of my cesspool of questions, doubts and decisions sounded wonderful. I especially anticipated the chance to spend five days in silence.

Several hundred people from all over the world had come to the Summer Solstice, as the event was called. The dry, pine and juniper-dotted hillsides of Espanola were colorful with vast tent cities. Bearded men in white leggings, shirts and turbans strolled the grounds. Women in white dresses and turbans carried white-clad babies. Children ran about, the boys with their never-cut hair turned up in a topknot on their heads.

I had brought my own tent and Leith and Todd shared one of their own. At four o'clock each morning the strains of guitars and chanting woke us as musicians strolled through the tent city calling us to morning meditation. This consisted of a long hour of sitting on the hard cement floor of a shaded, open-sided compound while prayers and chants were intoned. Then we could go to our tents to eat the bananas and oranges which had been dispensed to us at the previous day's evening meal.

There were lots of different activities one could choose from: yoga, nutrition, healing or face reading workshops, prayers, history, games, service--in which we offered our time to paint latrines, dining halls, etc. Every afternoon was reserved for Tantra Yoga. In these lengthy sessions, several hundred people sat cross-legged in long rows, men across from women, and intoned various chants and maintained prescribed postures while a venerable yogi leader directed us. I found the postures very difficult to maintain. For example, we might be directed to hold our arms in a prayer pose over our heads. Certain chants accompanied this pose, while we peered fixedly into the eyes of our partner. This could go on for 20 or 30 minutes while the yogi leader sat on a stage drinking tea.

The five days of silence, which I so eagerly anticipated, proved to be a disappointment. People could choose to participate in it or not. And we got into games of how we could communicate non-verbally --using writing pads, charades, miming ... Many, especially the children, had no part of the silence. The so-called silence seemed almost a joke, and I found it difficult to get myself into a place of honoring it.

I discovered, however, that the retreat offered me answers in a different way than I had expected. I was not so much attracted to interacting in the workshops or with the groups as I was attracted to the wild landscape. With the people preoccupied in their own activities, I had the freedom to walk and be alone on the extensive private grounds. I was at peace in the walking. I was aware of the integrity of the trees and the stones, of the ageless mountains and the sky, of the spirits of animals and the Indians who had moved through those juniper forests before me. I walked or sat quietly, having a sense, almost, of the guidance of the surrounding spirits funnelling into me. There were no lightning-striking messages from God. No meditative state of mind--but I felt peaceful and *some* Presence seemed to be there.

I used this quiet time to examine my situation. Some important awarenesses began to break through to my consciousness: *My life is only worth what comes from within myself. There are only external and temporary answers in careers and relationships and activities. The one way I will be in harmony and at peace and with some purpose is by being so within myself. No man, no job can give me the fulfillment I need. Perhaps temporarily, yes. But people die or change or leave. Jobs are lost or altered or I get sick and can't work. I can only be me through having a sense of wholeness and well-being within. How?*

Such overwhelming sadness filled me as I reviewed the last 10 to 13 years: years of living in turbid turmoil and anxiety and pressure, all in the superficial plane, hurrying here and there and taking no time to breathe or to be aware of my inner disharmony. Looking back, the overall picture was bleak--so full of activity, but so lacking in satisfaction. Always *dis*satisfied. Always striving, pushing and rushing. Always wanting the externals to be otherwise. Wanting Jack to be different. Wanting my business to be different. Wanting the raft trips to be different. Wanting the campfire musicians to play the guitar better. Wanting my body to be different. Rarely living in complete acceptance of what was in the moment.

Had I wasted those years? I couldn't believe that they had all been a waste. It certainly had taken me a long time to realize the degree of my disharmony. As if I had to live and relive the same superficialities and dissatisfactions before I could finally embark on change. *And AM I embarked on change?* I asked myself. *Am I, perhaps, too attached to comfort and laziness? Wouldn't it be nice to postpone transformation until it's more convenient?*

I wanted to be in the world with total inner harmony and strength, to be a participant and make a difference. Yet I didn't know how to do that. I wasn't in touch with my Source. I saw that there had to be a cleansing, opening, and willingness to let go: regarding relationships, the shop, the health problems, the allergies. All were places where I had to purge, to release. I had to let go of the food sensations which once so easily distracted, but only temporarily satisfied me. I had to let go of the illusion that a good man would bring out the real me, and that frantic toil in a shop would yield eventual fulfillment.

None of those had worked because I had been, and still was, incomplete, unfocused and continually searching for yet more and other answers. I had searched externally and that had proven to be dissatisfying. *The search must now go inward,* I told myself. I feared it, feared I was too undisciplined for the rigors of the journey. I feared I was attached to my lack of discipline and to my comfort. Perhaps I was attached to my search! To my dissatisfaction!

Taking a deep breath of the fragrant air, I looked up past the junipers toward the blue canopy of sky and said out loud, "Here I am, God, in New Mexico, and I'm ready for direction, for answers, for signals and messages. Send me a sign." But I knew that first I had to be open to WHATEVER came. And I was still working on that.

I was glad that I'd brought Leo Buscaglia's book, *Personhood*, with me to New Mexico. As I read his words, they spoke to my confusion, giving it significance and delineating purpose and meaning in the task ahead of me. He offered the comfort that others had trod this path before me, and he gave support and hope for the positive change I sought.

> *"It is only when we can no longer cope and fall under the pain and strain of nonfulfillment that we are forced to obtain some help or make some change. Usually this is just a token adjustment--vague and temporary--before we are returned to "real" life, as ill prepared as before."*
>
> *Leo Buscaglia,* ***Personhood***

I asked myself, *Am I prepared, at last, to move beyond token adjustments?*

As I anticipated the future, I felt hopeful. I thought that making the decision to embark on a new path, or more precisely, the acknowledgement that I was on this path willy nilly, would automatically yield splendid change. The health would magically improve, the wholesome people with whom I longed to associate would appear, the work and the finances would work out. It would be an exciting, stimulating, joyful journey--a release from all the old burdens that I carried. Little did I realize that it would appear to be the exact opposite--that I had much deeper water to wade through before the joy would come.

CHAPTER THREE

BACK IN PORTLAND from my Sikh sojourn, I was as mired as ever in the muck of making decisions about Bloomers, my flower shop. I knew I must get away from the business--whether by selling or leasing, I didn't yet know. I *did* know that I must study and grow in the area of self-knowledge, that I wanted to read, take classes and learn to meditate. I knew also that I needed to compile a resume although I had no idea where I might send it. And, I needed to sell the house so that Jack would have the money to move forward in his life. I hated the idea of losing my home, but it would unburden me of obligation and upkeep and give me the money to move forward also. But where?

Don't worry about the specifics! I told myself. *Ask only what I must do in the broad sense--so that I can move toward a life which affords the kind of thought, action and stimulation that I perceive in people like Frances Horn and Leo Buscaglia, a life where I exercise my intellect and my creativity.*

In New Mexico, and then back in Portland, it seemed that I kept encountering people who were leisurely and who enjoyed their lives--people who had fun, free-time activities and who lived without pressure. *How did they arrange that?* I wondered. Was it really possible to support oneself and still have play time? Time in which to move slowly, to spontaneously spend a night with a friend, or to relax in a hot tub? *Of course it's possible,* I told myself. *I just haven't tried it, and I have to learn, just as I had to learn how to walk.*

Two weeks after returning from New Mexico, it seemed that my body was improving. Then Kabang! Everything fell apart. I wanted to scream, the pain from the buttocks down my legs was so penetrating. I kept reminding myself that it had diminished other times. Yet I couldn't understand why the pain attacked again, and in different ways. Why was I not better in such a way that I didn't slip backwards at the least little alteration in the status quo?

I wanted only to move and be energetic, to lead a "normal" life. My body repeatedly told me, "No--that is not to be." I longed to talk to someone, to express my fear, sorrow and pain. Yet when I had inflicted those expressions on my few friends, it yielded no real help for me and just boredom for them.

I yearned to eat something sweet--cookies, dates, or at least a bite of fruit. Even a piece of bread would have been ambrosial. Everything I craved, however, was either high carbohydrate or allergic--poison for my body. I was sick of eating vegetables for breakfast, lunch and dinner. The only taste thrill I got was from almond butter or nuts, lots of fats, but I knew that was overloading. So I felt guilty if I did eat and deprived if I didn't.

I wanted to accomplish so much. I wanted to attend outings with friends. I wanted to practice songs with my singing partner and good friend, Carol, at night. I wanted to work in my beautiful garden. Yet I felt drained; the buttock pain persisted even when I was standing up or lying on my stomach.

There had been times earlier that summer when I had been a dynamo of fun and energy. And then there were times such as this when I was exhausted, drained, discouraged; allowed, it seemed, to live only in pain, with the tantalizing joys and glories of the outer world still not mine to reach for. No carefree singles life, no spontaneous tumbles in the sack with men. No heady, hard-core workouts on the racquetball court, no long days of hiking or of sweaty yard work. No pushing of my body at all. I was realizing the truth of Leo Buscaglia's words: *"Pain is truly a great instigator for change."*

Am I not allowed to venture back into the world? I lamented. *Is there some force telling me I must continue to renounce taking pleasure in externals: in sex, fun, people, activities, in my lovely house and yard, and in simply sitting in the sun on a Saturday?*

I felt so helpless, so unable to do the right thing. I thought I had been listening to my inner voice and that even in the midst of the past months' myriad activities, that I was staying aware and in touch and was growing. *Patience!* I told myself. *But I want relief now!* And I thought, *Who am I kidding? Have I really been open to change?* In fact, I had kept trying to go back to my high-pressured, frantic and physical behaviors, but the pain wouldn't let me. I *had* gotten better before. I was determined that I would again! I just hadn't expected to backslide. *Is this going to be the eternal pattern,* I wondered, *until I give up everything?*

I felt utterly alone in my pain. I longed to be held and comforted. Yet I knew that was unrealistic. Even when Jack was living with me, I had still felt alone in my anguish.

I thought of rakish and handsome Sam, the man with whom I'd been having a slight fling, and I knew that he couldn't possibly empathize with my situation. He had no desire to be involved with a woman on such a level. "Sam's problem," my brother had once told me, "is that way down deep he's shallow." Sam's idea was: Keep it light. Keep it fun. Keep it active. No negatives or turmoils. At least not with casual friends. Maybe once the relationship became closer or deeper. But that wasn't what he wanted. Nor did I--with him. Yet I would have liked a friend in such low times.

The words from Leo Buscaglia's book, *Personhood*, sustained me:

> *"Continuous growth is dependent upon some source of discomfort and .... the degree of change is positively related to the degree of pain. Pain is a very human way of demanding change."*

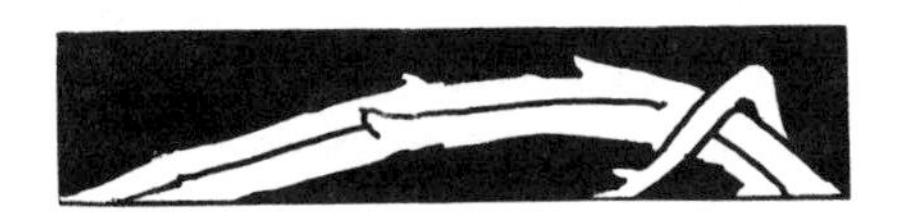

CHAPTER FOUR

THE DAY CAME in early August when my naturopath, Dr. Henin, said, "We must determine whether or not it's multiple sclerosis." I nearly fell off my chair and my stomach twisted into 200 knots. I'd gone through a lot of fear of MS the year before, when the symptoms first hit me. Now it was cropping up again. I thought, *What if it is?* And then, *What if it **isn't**?* Much as I dreaded it being MS, there was a certain part of me that said, *There you see! It really exists. It's not in my head. I'm not running after exotic diseases, being led on by crazy doctors.*

How terrible to want to have a label, dreadful as it might be, just so that I could be taken seriously by those around me. My pain and anguished behavior would then be legitimized, and the limits that I had to live in would be understood by others--and by me. That was certainly a "wrong view" if ever there was one.

Part of me was determined that this was not MS and that, in fact, it was just a very unglamorous and inexplicable allergy/candida problem that was difficult to identify and resolve. Actually, the label didn't matter insofar as what existed. No matter what it was called, I had certain out-of-whack systems.

I expected that I was going to have to do a lot of giving up of food and a lot of work to reclaim my body. *I welcome it!* I told myself. *I can do it! I have to trust that it's nothing more than the candida. I've just overdone the cheating on my diet. Face up to the literally distasteful task of simply dealing straightforwardly with it. No fun and games. No more cheating. No going along with the crowd.*

Serious, down-to-basics restrictions. But they'll be worth it.

The next morning as I walked in the warm sun, I was plagued by alternating sensations of weakness, numbness, achiness, soreness, pinched feelings. *But at least I can walk!* I kept repeating. *I am determined that this is the worst I will be. I am making lots of changes. From here on out, it's nothing but better and better!*

Dr. Henin managed to schedule me for some blood tests and to see Dr. Swank, a leading national authority on MS, at the Oregon Health Sciences University. Dr. Henin must have pulled a few strings, because my appointment was scheduled for within two weeks. Usually Dr. Swank was booked up six months in advance.

The blood takers at Providence Hospital were very nice. They explained that for the MS test the blood doesn't travel well, which was why I had to come to the hospital. There was some kind of protein substance which showed up in the blood of MS people and was absent from the blood of other people.

The blood man said, "How lucky for you that you are self-employed because then you can allow yourself rest periods. Dr. Swank puts people on a two hour a day rest schedule."

Boy, oh, boy! What a joke! Two hours a day! Me! Immediately I wondered, *How on earth am I going to go about applying for jobs where I have to be alert, learn, rise to occasions and work steady hours?* How fortunate I'd been in the past weeks, owning my own business and being able to go home or to the doctor whenever I needed to--which had been daily.

I took stock of my options, getting down to the basic questions:

Q: *What is the worst possible thing that could happen?*

A: *I'll just close up the shop and walk away.*

(Well, squeaked this frightened little voice, that's not so awful.)

Q: *How will I live?*

A: *I'll sell the shares Dad gave me years ago and live on that while I heal. I can learn to do at-home things--weddings--writing--massage??? I'm sure Mom and Dad will help me if necessary.*

Money, I acknowledged, was the very least of my worries. I knew that I could turn to the one source that always supported and loved me--Mom and Dad. Perhaps that was the key to all of the dis-ease. The big need for love and support.

In spite of my parents' material assistance over the years, in many ways I'd felt unloved and unsupported. Even if that was not the truth, that was the way I felt. A new thought struck me. Although I detested the idea, I couldn't help wondering, *Since I have difficulty asking for anything overtly, maybe I am subconsciously thinking that I'll get help if I'm in a condition where I obviously cannot get it for myself.* If that was the case then, clearly, I had to change the negatives that I'd programmed throughout my mind and body. I had to learn to accept my own goodness, abilities, lovingness, vulnerabilities, my own need to ask.

I decided that I could no longer postpone acting differently. Initiating my first attempt in asking for help, I phoned my friend, Peter. When I first met Peter Dane three years earlier, I'd been attracted by his almost blase', bearded good looks and gentle, open manner. A skilled massage therapist and counselor, Peter had given me my first massage. It had been like a revelation--the first opening up to the connection of my brain with my, until then, distantly-related body.

Gradually, Peter had become a friend, the first man with whom I could express my confusions, doubts, and yearnings toward intimacy, passion, and inner growth. We became lovers, but we each also had marriage partners. Amidst strained feelings and confusions, we slowly diminished our ties. During the last year's difficulties, I'd avoided turning to Peter for his counseling skills--fearing that he might misconstrue my motives--fearing he'd think I wanted the emotional involvement of the past resurrected. Now, though, I realized, *It is time for me to learn to step beyond that. To release the fears of being rejected or misunderstood. To know that I am a good person and that I can take charge of attending to my needs no matter what the outer world might think or what it might do.*

> *"That's what life-changing is--learning. When something isn't going well in your life, you can learn something new. You can* ***teach yourself*** *what you need."*
>
> *Read and Rusk,* ***I Want to Change, But I Don't Know How***

That evening, as I sat outside and watched the sundown shadows lengthen on the flower-filled patio, I felt a glow of satisfaction. I could be proud of myself that day. I had broken some old habits. Rather than hurrying off to work in the morning, I had stopped in at my favorite bookstore, where I read books and listened to inspirational tapes for two hours. Instead of pushing myself to keep going, I came home and rested when I was tired. I recognized the need to be with a friend who could help me, and I had gone ahead and called Peter for an appointment. I even left my name on his answer machine. All those risks! He might think I was chasing him! His *wife* might think I was chasing him! But I took the risk. Smiling inwardly, I mentally patted myself on the back. At last I was choosing the path that was right for me--instead of acting so as to meet someone else's expectations.

Another big pat on the back! I had eaten mono-foods (one food at a time) all day--tracking my reactions: Green pepper for breakfast; mid-morning, carrots; later some rice; chicken for lunch; mid-afternoon, celery juice; at night, a big bowl of broccoli. I had eaten no fat at all and almost no carbohydrates. The result was that I felt good, not bloated or heavy or full--actually a little light and lean. And there had been no lightheadedness or other reactions to any of the foods.

I smiled as I remembered how the day before I had initiated yet another unfamiliar behavior. I had donned my beautiful, new, silky and lacy lingerie. What a change from my usual practical T-shirt and from the old Barbara who once would have blushed to admit an interest in such obviously male-fetching apparel. But I *enjoyed* me in it. I enjoyed feeling feminine and beautiful and looking at myself in it. True, it would have been nice to share, but since there was no man, I still could enjoy the total pleasure for myself.

I was also learning much from my continued reading of Tom Rusk and Randy Read's book, *I Want to Change, But I Don't Know How*. I learned that I had not loved myself. I needed to practice self-love. Stepping inside the house, I stood before the mirror and attempted to look at myself with detachment. *There is Barbara,* I said. *What do I see? A tired, careworn face; blue eyes; shag of brown hair, somewhat sun-bleached; medium height; a symmetrical body--at 114 pounds the slimmest it's ever been, but flabbier.*

What do I like about her? I asked the reflection. *She is nice, sensitive, responsible, caring, efficient, funny. What don't I like? She is selfish, doesn't listen completely to people, doesn't do as much as she could to be a friend to her friends or to show love to those she loves.*

Leaving the mirror, and returning to the patio, I said to myself, *Try these new phrases on for size: I love myself. I am a good person. I am willing to risk, to change. Willing to let go of obsolete and negative thought patterns. Willing to open up myself and my body with loving thoughts, habits and actions.*

I remembered a phrase I'd read at the bookstore that afternoon: *"Only those who dare, truly love."* That was my task, to *dare* to act in accordance with *my* needs and desires. Only then would I truly love--first myself and then others.

The next morning I awoke keyed up with nervousness in anticipation of my impending meeting with Peter. I also woke up with my hands and arms tingling just as they had done the year before. *Oh, no! Not this too!* I tried to keep from panicking. I meditated as best I could. I kept remembering, *It **does** go away.*

Sitting that afternoon in Peter's office in his house, I expressed everything. My awareness of my ability to heal myself. The fear that I wouldn't. My recognition that the only people who would take care of me were Mom and Dad. That I had come to Peter for support and love, yet I felt uncomfortable because I was asking for it as a paying customer. He decided to divorce himself from therapist and become just friend.

"What do you need?" he asked.

"Love and support."

"What would feel good?"

"To be held."

I answered it all and I asked for exactly what I needed. No beating around the bush anymore! As a result, my needs were satisfied and we both shared the best exchange we'd had in a long time.

Much as I wanted only to retreat home and rest and read after leaving Peter's, I felt good enough to go to the shop. *Better work while I have the energy,* I thought. Once there, it was odd almost, how receptive and conversational I was with Tauni, my sweet young manager. How unusual it was for me to join her in joking around, and simply not worry about the lack of sales or what was going to become of everything.

I kept telling myself, *It will all work out. I can make no decisions and no plans until after my appointment with Dr. Swank next week. Then I will know how my life is to change and what I have to do.*

The next evening, Wendy, a breezy young photographer whom I'd met at the Chamber of Commerce, came over with her new camera to photograph the cats. She took lots of shots out on the patio of me holding first one squirming cat and then another. I was pleased to at last capture some memory of my loyal little housemates. Woo's grey fur had fluffed and puffed out handsomely and he no longer sported the fierce Chinese opera face that originally prompted me to name him Chi Wu. Betty, dear little calico queen, with her six-toed catcher's mitt feet, was curious, preening, and tolerant. The patriarch of my little trio, Gherkin, had already undergone his share of photo sessions in past years, so he was spared such indignities.

Wendy stayed on for steaks and we had a fine, fun time joking and sharing. As she got ready to leave, she said how nice it had been and, "You're sure funny."

Isn't that funny! I thought. It was true. To all appearances, my whole life was crashing, yet I was really "on," and even though I was tired, I rose to the occasion and enjoyed it thoroughly. I thought to myself, *Perhaps I* ***am*** *changing. I* ***choose*** *to be happy, strong, witty and funny, loving and sharing.* It had been a delightful evening. I did nothing physical, but I still had fun!

After Wendy left, I turned off the lights and sat quietly in my living room. Silver streaks of moonlight streamed through the skylights and the uncurtained windows bathing the room in a friendly brightness. *I* ***am*** *beating this thing!* I told myself. *I resolve to lead a "normal" life. Perhaps it will not be as physically active as before, but today has shown me how there are wonderful people available to me. There* ***will*** *be more delightful days and people!* It seemed paradoxical. I was living with pain and with very much uncertainty. Yet I was calm, and I even enjoyed love.

"Pain, you see is power. Pain can paralyze or it can motivate. It can help you find the courage necessary to overcome ***fear*** *and* ***habit****."*

Read and Rusk, ***I Want to Change, But I Don't Know How***

CHAPTER FIVE

THE NEXT DAY I didn't go to work at all. Why should I? I continued reading the book on how to change. "If what you're doing now isn't working, do something different." I knew my body needed rest. My mind needed rest. So I took the plunge and did something "different." I stayed at home. Yet I couldn't help worrying about where the line was crossed from taking care of myself to shirking responsibility.

All will work out, I kept telling myself. *All that I need comes to me. I can live on my shares, or Mom and Dad can help out if need be.* The time had come to overcome my adherence to everyone else's rules, which said that it was *bad* to accept help from one's parents; that there was only virtue in making it on one's own. It was time to choose *my* path--to do what was right for *me*. The words to the song continually reminded me;

"Whether I'm right, or whether I'm wrong, I've got to be me."
from, ***I've Got to be Me***

I found it quite surprising that I could have myriad, strange body symptoms and still have days of pleasantness. I kept my exertions to the household things only--thankful that I had the energy to at least do those. I continually told myself that I could trust that the pain *would* go away and I'd once again be able to play racquetball, stretch, jog or work in the yard. What if I couldn't? What if that didn't happen? There *were* alternatives. But could I live with them?

Two mornings later I was on my way out the door to a Louise Hay Healing Seminar when someone called to say it had been cancelled. Suddenly I found myself at the start of a sparkling, sunny day and it was completely free. I wanted to do something reviving--something for me. Something different. I decided to drive out to Sauvie Island on the Columbia River and walk.

Within the hour I was ambling along the rustic rolling roads of Sauvie Island. Walking wasn't an automatic response. I had to mentally conjure up the movement and the energy. Stiff, tender, achy, my legs responded as if they had crampy clumps of muscles with lead weights on them. Negotiating the slight hills was the hardest. Sometimes my hands and arms began to tingle. Yet I was walking! That was an accomplishment.

And what a place to walk. The island was pristine, so unaffected by the proximity of Portland. No fast food blemishes or gas stations, no sign boards or souvenir shops marred its rustic splendor. Just farms and farm houses and the long, oaty grasses and colorful summer weeds and flowers blooming along the narrow roadways. Houses and fields were well tended. Nothing looked junky, as so often occurs in rural areas.

Returning to my car, I decided to drive to the nude beach. Why not, as long as I was so close already, and I was prepared with my folding chair, towel and books? I felt very clever knowing just where I wanted to go--the same place my friend and I had lazed one sunny afternoon. The spacious, sandy spot was somewhat secluded, set at the very end of the designated nude area and broken up by trees and grasses. Pitching my gear, I shed my clothes without even a thought and settled in to read and enjoy the sun. All so simple and natural as if I'd done it dozens of times, instead of just once before.

In the evening, although I was tired and my legs felt stiff and weak, my spirits were high. Despite my difficulties, I had found meaning, fulfillment and pleasure in the day. I had walked. I was maintaining my muscle tone. I felt good, too, with my continuing practice of eating foods one at a time as I tried to establish safe and unsafe ones.

Throughout the day, as on other days, as I drove, walked, or prepared food, I enlisted even my singing as a form of inspiration. Banished were the mournful Irish lyrics with melodies so well suited to my soprano voice. I sang, instead, the bright, up, positive words that reinforced how I wanted to see myself:

> *"Hey! Look me over! Lend me an ear,*
> *Fresh out of clover and mortgaged up to here,*
> *But don't pass the plate folks,*
> *Don't pass the buck,*
> *I figure whenever you're down and out,*
> *the only way is up!"*
>
> *From the musical,* ***Wildcat***

My reading of *I Want To Change, But I Don't Know How* brought up the question: WHAT NEED DOES ILLNESS SUPPLY FOR ME? If I honestly answered, there were two big needs:

1. *The need to learn to say "no."*

Already I was using the illness as an excuse not to do certain things. It was an excuse not to write to a family member. On the phone one night, instead of honestly telling that person, "I don't care to write to you," I said, "My body's not up to it."

The illness gave me an excuse to stay away from work, to say "no" to the shop. As if I could close the doors and no one could say, "She failed." It would all be because of my health.

Obviously, I needed to learn how to say "no" *without guilt* to the events, people and pressures that dragged on my well-being,

2. *The need to ask for what I needed.*

Illness gave me a legitimate reason to ask people for help. I could see myself telling my landlord that I had MS and expected that maybe he'd give me a break on the rent, find me a smaller shop, and not reject my requests for help. Illness also made it okay to ask Mom and Dad for financial assistance. After all, a sick person wasn't expected to have to make it on their own. Now maybe Jack would mow the lawn or cut wood for me and I wouldn't feel like a pest for asking him.

On top of those payoffs was the fact that feeling bad physically diminished my interest and need for sex, so I didn't feel left out sexually. And, besides, if I were ill, maybe Tauni would decide not to look for another job and would agree to stay and work longer for me.

How true were those points? Surely the negatives of being ill outweighed the advantages!

I also asked myself, WHAT AM I LEARNING FROM ILLNESS?

1. *Being ill gives me purpose, a challenge, something to become, the goal of health to be strived for.*
2. *It forces me to take stock of myself, my life--honestly.*

So--I had needs! Such an idea had never before occurred to me. Clearly, my major needs had not been met during the last years. I needed love, but I had lacked love--of self and from others. I needed purpose, self-respect, a sense of worth, fun. I needed security--to know that my needs could be met.

"When you're missing something, your hurting says, "Wake up!"
*Read and Rusk, **I Want to Change, But I Don't Know How***

My reading and self-scrutiny forced me to realize some important truths about how I'd chosen to behave throughout my life. I'd done things so that I'd receive approval--with the result that I became a slave to other people's definitions. I always thought that I had courage--emigrating to Australia when I was 22, teaching school there with no training, hitch-hiking across continents, building my own business, singing publicly--but in many ways I hadn't. During my marriage I'd avoided speaking out to Jack fearing I'd hurt him. When I'd been involved with Peter, I wouldn't ask him outright what was the status of our relationship. I'd not had the courage to communicate honestly--with my family, with customers, with friends, and with men in particular.

Although I hadn't been afraid to hitchhike around the world, I had other fears. I had been fearful of failing in other people's eyes (Dad's, Mom's, Jack's, customers', racquetball partners' ...), fearful of not holding up my responsibilities to them or of not receiving their approval. And now I was fearful of not holding up my responsibility to myself, to my body and its healing. The words of Royal Robbins, the mountain climber, spoke to the place in which I found myself:

"You will never know how much you can do until you extend yourself to your limit, and you don't know that until you fall trying."

As a young woman whenever I read books about concentration camp survivors and others who had endured terrible hardships, I used to think, "Thank goodness I don't have to go through what they did." And I always feared that I'd not have the courage to endure dire circumstances. Now, I saw that I'd not lived even my daily humdrum life with courage.

Courage was the choice to be vulnerable. Courage was what I manifested when I plunged into life. It was when I took the risk of phoning a man in regard to his offhand treatment of me, regardless of how he might respond. Courage was what I felt when I risked looking silly, being misconstrued or rejected, or having people angry at me. Now, as I started mustering the courage to take such risks, I noticed that it really felt good!

Courage was choice. *"The valiant at least pause, agonize the alternatives, then choose,"* said Reed and Rusk in *I Want to Change, But I Don't Know How*. As I faced the difficult decisions and choices before me, I realized that there was the possibility that I might pick "wrong." But only if I courageously faced the decisions could I hope to come to freedom from fears, freedom from tyranny.

This made sense, and yet it was so difficult to truly accept and put it into practice. I felt that I was undergoing a heavy lesson in developing my courage--through no great initiative or outreach of my own. Life's circumstances had thrown me at it. There was just no choice but to be courageous. I knew all too well that I had only myself to rely upon. But there was a paradox in that. For, when I took the responsibility of relying on myself and looking after myself, I wound up acting in ways that brought me the people, support and situations that I needed.

"Some obstacles," declared Reed and Rusk, "are so high or so thick, that we can't surmount them by calm choice. It takes determination, dedication, or perhaps the moral equivalent of war." I felt that I was going into battle to reclaim my Self; to renew my faith in myself, my courage, initiative, and sense of self-worth; my belief in who I was. I hadn't sought this battle, and yet here I was.

> *"If thou will not fight thy battle of life because in selfishness thou art afraid of the battle, thy resolution is in vain: nature will compel thee."*
>
> **Bhagavad Gita**, *18;59*

CHAPTER SIX

AUGUST FOURTEENTH, MY D-Day, arrived. Dr. Henin accompanied me into the cluttered cubbyhole of Dr. Swank's office deep in the bowels of the Oregon Health Sciences University. I fidgeted with nervousness and the jelly-like weakness in my legs was the worst it had ever been.

Dr. Swank was a world-reknowned authority on MS. For over thirty years, he had conducted on-going studies of MS patients, starting at the University of Montreal and then continuing in Oregon. He had developed a blood test that showed up certain irregularities in individuals with MS. There was also an eye flicker test that helped positively identify MS people. The stickler was that although a positive test result was, indeed, an indication of MS, a negative result was not necessarily proof that a person was MS-free. Frequently, people who tested negatively from one year to the next, actually displayed very definite MS symptoms.

Dr. Swank tested my eyes, then my neurological responses and my balance. Finally he said "The tests do not show that you have MS. But the tests are never definitive. I'm 90% sure you've got it. You are arresting it early. If you follow the diet, relieve your stress, avoid overdoing, you can lead a normal life."

I thought to myself, *Isn't that desirable anyway, ill or not???*

The main thing I wanted to know was, what could *I* do to reverse this? I bombarded Dr. Swank with questions about MS and about my options. His answers gave me hope, for I saw that, yes, there *were* things that I could do.

From his studies, Dr. Swank explained, he had determined that there was a correlation between high fat intake and incidences of MS. He had tracked patients for 20 or 30 years who had been on his low-fat diet, and the success rate was remarkable. There had actually been a 95% rate of remission in those who stuck to the diet. Patients usually remained wherever they were physically at the time they began the diet, but some patients had even improved. Sometimes, though, patients were pretty crippled before they got onto the diet, and in those cases it was less successful.

Leaning across his desk, Dr. Swank handed me a huge notebook which was crammed with four years of his MS newsletters. I was also given a set of diet sheets to fill out every day. Their purpose was to help me monitor my fat intake. I, who loved fats, was about to cut nearly every vestige of them from my diet.

Dr. Swank differentiated between fats and oils. Fats were anything that was saturated or that became solid in the refrigerator. Therefore, all dairy products, hydrogenated margarines and coconut were off the list. As was red meat and certain fatty fish and the dark meat of poultry. It was important, however, to get the essential oils into the body because they seemed to be precursors for the building of a healthy myelin sheaf (the part of the nerves that breaks down in MS). Certain desirable components made up these essential oils in varying amounts. The most desirable of all oils was evening primrose oil. But it cost $58 for a little bottle. The next most desirable configuration was found in cod liver oil. I was instructed to take four "C.L.O" perls daily--the equivalent of one teaspoon of liquid.

With a sinking feeling, I listened as Dr. Swank told me, "You will have to limit your fat intake to ten teaspoons of oils and three teaspoons of fats a day." He gave me a sheet on which he had compiled the equivalents. I could refer to the sheet and see that one egg equaled one teaspoon of FAT, a can of drained tuna equaled one teaspoon of OIL and 15 almonds equaled one teaspoon of OIL, etc.

Dr. Swank stressed the importance of resting for two hours in the middle of the day. *How on earth will I carry that off?* I wondered. I cringed as Dr. Swank said, "No racquetball, no competitive sports, no jogging unless you've built up to it over time."

Before my appointment, I'd come to a decision about what I must do. No matter what Dr. Swank told me, I knew I needed time to rest.

I planned to give myself six months or so to really relax, rest, relieve stress and build up my strength. Then I would start challenging myself a little bit at a time. I'd take on no full-time job, just part-time.

It sounded wonderful--six months to rest! *I* had control. I could *choose* wellness, restfulness and non-stress, could choose to love myself and to give myself the support I needed and deserved. It was a choice: to take control of my life, and to face my humanity squarely.

Making the choice was the first step, but actualizing it was not so simple. I would be many months into the process before I was able to relax my judgments about my inability to fulfill my decision. I wouldn't have needed to change if I'd been so completely together that I could simply decide--and act.

At home after seeing Dr. Swank, I started to plan for the future. In regard to the business, I phoned my landlord. He was available at four o'clock. So there was no time to gather more than a little nervousness. I had always felt apologetic about taking up the busy man's time. But now things were different. I was nervous, but I gave myself permission to succeed or fail, to present my program as best I could and if it wasn't "perfect," well, I was only human. When we met, I took my time, saying what I wanted to say instead of forgetting important details in my haste to race through to the finish and relieve the important man of my humble presence. He said, "I'm sorry to see you pull out. The shop has been a colorful attraction. I'd like to see you hang on."

He promised to phone me the following week and to let me know if he could help me by reducing the rent or by giving me a smaller shop space. There would be more days of waiting for answers.

The next morning I saw Dr. Henin. We talked for two hours about my healing program. He listened with compassion to my fears, answered my questions, and laid everything on the line: the importance of the diet, the differences between the fats and the oils, the best way to exercise, the necessity of rest. One thing he said pleased me, which was that since I was now dealing with MS, I might as well cut out the nystatin (a yeast killing drug) and the candida diet. Suddenly my world opened up! Fruit! Soy sauce! Vinegar! Flavors I'd been missing for so long. If I could eat more of those foods, then eliminating the fats seemed less awful.

After leaving Dr. Henin's, I gave myself the gift of the day, allowing myself the luxury of roaming through the quaint shops of Portland's Yamhill Market. At home I read in the sun, and then, with the Walkman symphony, I set out upon my neighborhood loop. As I willed each leg to move forward, I thought about my day. To all appearances I had been a normal person, walking around town, driving, trying on clothes, ordering my piano music. *This isn't so bad,* I told myself. *I am committed to continuing to support and love this person, Barbara. I give her compassion and applaud her courage to lead life on her own path.* I was proud of myself for at last choosing to wear my bathing suit top with my shorts out walking. I could say, *Who cares what the one or two people I pass think? I choose* ***my*** *path--what's best for me.*

"Whether I'm right, or whether I'm wrong,
Whether I find a place in this world,
or never belong,
I've Got to be Me! I've Got to be Me!
Who else can I be but what I am?"
from, ***I've Got to be Me***

Even though I wanted to learn all I could about the MS experience, I chose not to get involved with the MS society. Whether or not it would have been helpful, I don't know. It struck me that joining the MS society would be another way of reinforcing my identity as a victim of the disease. So I stayed away. I sought out the people who had been successful in changing their circumstances of disease. I interviewed anyone who had overcome MS, cancer, or any other sickness. Their improvement spurred me to believe that I, too, could be successful.

A few days after my appointment with Dr. Swank, my new friend, Wendy, introduced me to Mrs. Davis, a woman who had endured MS for twenty years. She opened my eyes to the hard realities of MS. "You get very weak and tired. You are not reliable. You work within your limits. You don't do the things that you used to do, at least not to the degree you did them. You rest. You get rid of the stress. The stress is what pulls you down. Once you lose your nerve function, you don't get it back. You use the support of the people who love you to keep yourself up. You eliminate the people who don't or won't support you, as they're very detrimental. You follow the diet, which is the pits. Sometimes you want to scream and you get stuck. Then you get the people around you to help you up. The stresses are the things! You can do well if you keep the stress down."

Mrs. Davis was about to get her first wheelchair. She did less and less of what she used to do. Yet, even with a wheel chair, she was flying to England in a month. At least the world did not end. One could still travel, albeit in a wheelchair.

After talking with Mrs. Davis, I realized more than ever the absurdity of my going to work. It was too much. It took more out of me and killed off what reserves I had left. As I had done so often for the last year, I asked myself, *How do I extricate myself from this shop?* Turning to my network system, I phoned different friends. They weren't home. At last I reached Dave and, later, Leith, in Phoenix. They gave me love and the reassurance I needed. "Yes," they agreed, "the business is only dollars. Your health is priceless. It's okay to just kill the business off. Only one goal, one obligation exists: that is to yourself."

I continued to wrestle with the decision about the shop, but I couldn't quite step over the line. Despite the encouragement from Leith and Dave, I still felt keyed up and anxious about what to do. On one particularly anguish-filled day, I once again phoned my local network: Wendy, Lori, Marilyn. My most loyal customer, Ann, agreed to oversee the shop for as long as might be necessary. Gradually, my tense, achy body calmed down, and with relaxation came a discernable difference in its energy and mobility.

That afternoon I decided that there was no harm in asking for that which would help me the most, and I gathered my courage and wrote to Mom and Dad asking for money. That would take the financial pressures off and get me through indefinitely until such time as I had the energy to support myself. Taking one more step in asking for help, I rang Carol, my most staunch supporter, and asked her if she would be able to drive me places. Driving had become terribly taxing. My legs were so weak that I could hardly hold down the gas pedal. It seemed as if I was asking, asking, asking. How could I receive all this help and not hold up my end? This was strange territory.

When I was just sitting or lying down I felt fine. I was warm and comfortable on my patio, surrounded by the cheery flowers and the lush green umbrella of the trees. I tried not to think about how it would be to be alone and cold in the winter months with no flowers and no leaves.

Looking ahead to six months of not working seemed like a vacation, but it also hung over me oppressively. There were no men at all who would be calling on me or phoning or to whom I could turn for help with the maintenance and repairs of the house and yard. Mostly, there were no men to relate to, to care about me. But I'd been single before--until I was twenty-eight--and survived.

As I embarked on my time alone, I thought, *I wish I could believe that there will be relationships. My ability to interact is so limited. How many days will go by with only the cats for a loving touch?*

In the depths of my isolation, I couldn't begin to guess the unimagined quality of the relationships that would eventually unfold. As I restyled the quality of my relationship to myself, that change would one day be reflected in the men and women who I began to attract into my life.

Alone, sitting in my woodsy patio or in my wood-stained house with its high beam ceilings, skylights and big windows, I was surrounded by pretty things and material comfort. Yet my body was a constant bundle of *dis*comfort. The future, my only hope, weighed heavily. I wondered, *Will I, too, need a wheelchair when I am 60, like Mrs. Davis?*

I grew up with the message that people with money or creature comforts suffered, like Rockefeller with all his millions only being able to eat mush--or something like that. I wondered if I was sending myself a message that as long as I had money, things, material well-being, I somehow deserved to be ill? Was I perpetuating this message by stopping work and being willing to rely on Mom and Dad for financial support for several months?

Well, I thought, *at least I've found a purpose in life: to rise above this disease, to transcend the pitfalls that seek to entrap me, to make a worthwhile life out of the hand that I've been dealt.* Yet, I also asked myself, *If my purpose is to heal, then wouldn't the act of becoming healed nullify that purpose?* Something else, I realized, would have to step into that void. And I still wonder how many of us, identifying with our purpose--of healing, rising above, conquering, defeating some obstacle, whether it's illness, jobs or tyrants--actually prolong that process because we cannot abide being once again without purpose?

I saw the upcoming six months alone as very necessary. As a time for no external distractions. A time for coming into touch with Barbara and for learning to know her and to love her. *What a task!* I thought. *How strange that it is only now, at age 39, that I am starting to come to grips with loving myself!* How sad that it should be so, and that it should be so difficult. How sad, too, that I spent years denying my needs, suppressing self-love, directing all my energy to diffusing my positives. But now, a new tide was rising.

So I retreated, keeping at bay resentments and impatience. *It's only for a while and for a special time,* I told myself. *But I can come back, and when I do I'll be even more the special person into which I am evolving. No wheel chair! No canes! Normal life within limits for me! I've got what it takes!*

> *"There are really only two ways to approach life--as victim or as gallant fighter--and you must decide if you want to act or react, deal your own cards or play with a stacked deck. And if you don't decide which way to play with life, it always plays with you."*
>
> *Merle Shain, from* ***Each Day a New Beginning***

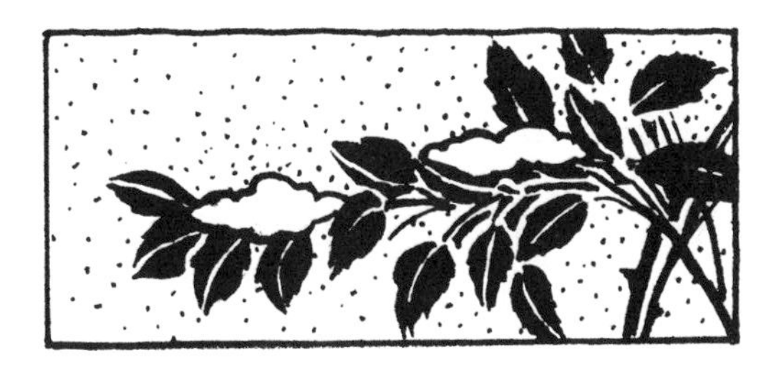

CHAPTER SEVEN

JAN PAUL, IN whose vision seminar I participated two years earlier, stopped by. He was an attractive, intelligent, very intuitive Frenchman, and he asked questions which made me think.

"What are you going to do in these six months?"

"Change old habits."

"How?"

"Change behavior. Make a concerted effort."

"Haven't you always been making a concerted effort?"

This question brought me up short for, after all, it seemed that the past few years had been a deluge of effort. Yet look where I was.

He said, "You are a people pleaser--also a controller, and very good at slipping from one mode to the other. ... What is your body telling you?"

"To stop doing, doing, doing."

He looked knowingly at me, "You are in a tremendous position for finding out about yourself. ... This is your time to just be with Barbara. How will you do that?"

I told him what I'd been envisioning, "To meditate. Read. Walk. Sing. I know I must avoid distractions. It's so easy, even now, to be tempted to do, do, do."

He assured me, "You *can* make your body whole. You *can* support yourself. You *can* be successful, it's all about loving yourself. You wonder what it is that people want back from you. They just want you to be you. They want the person who is you to shine out and share with them."

In the past I'd often wondered, why were people nice to me? Why did they help me? The wondering arose from my own inability to love myself. If *I* didn't love Barbara, then I certainly couldn't expect others to. If I didn't think Barbara deserved help, then how could I expect others to offer it? Yet in spite of that, some people did love and some did help. Now I realized that Barbara was a person whom I *could* love and for whom I could feel compassion and whose needs were worthy of being met. It was going to be very interesting to see how I proceeded in the next six months!

The next day I was sitting on the patio feeling lonely and sorry for myself. Recognizing what had brought on my bout of self pity, I knew that there was something important that I had to do. It was to make a giant leap ahead of myself and go beyond comparing. I asked myself, *So what if I can't hike up a mountain, with or without a heavy pack? So what if I can't do the aerobics and have the lean legs?* For the moment, those were other people's paths, but not mine. I had to cross over to accepting and enjoying and finding the value in my own path. Barbara's path. What was right for me. "It's not what we are, it's what we do with it," Jan Paul had told me.

I didn't want to be sad, and I especially didn't want to show it. Yet the sadness surfaced. My thoughts turned to my stone entry stairs, and I mentally figured how I would have to alter the house if I ever got a wheelchair. That time would mean perhaps even further letting go. Goodbye to the house and the patio. *So what if it happens?* I asked myself. *I'm on a journey which is carrying me toward my self, to self-power, to self-healing, to self-effectiveness. I learn daily the art of loving myself, and I:*

> *"use my discomfort to give myself the courage to* ***risk living*** *in more satisfying ways."*
>
> *Read and Rusk,* ***I Want to Change, But I Don't Know How***

I savored the blessed warm days with flowers and birds and cats sprawled belly-up to keep cool. But winter was coming. *Instead of dreading the winter,* I wrote in my journal, *I can anticipate it for the new, unknown people and circumstances that will be opening up for me, and for the better health and strength that I* ***know*** *will be developing.*

I remember the inner tug of war as I made myself talk or write in positive, rather than negative, terms about the loss of summer and the approaching winter. Every time I chose to speak in a way that expressed acceptance of what was so, I reinforced my ability to be in a mode of openness to seeing that, indeed, there were positives in all things.

In another way I appreciated the solitude. I couldn't imagine negotiating my dietary or physical problems with someone around, couldn't imagine Jack or anyone else preparing meals or caring to deal with the difficulties of my diet and my restrictions. I knew that if we'd still been living together and Jack wasn't helping me, I'd have felt nothing but resentment and abandonment. Even having someone as understanding as my dear friend Carol would have been difficult for me to deal with. I'd have hated so much to have to rely on her help, and I felt I couldn't expend the energy required to be pleasant and conversational.

Despite the times when I felt terribly isolated, on the whole, it seemed easier to be alone. There was so much to learn about my emerging way of being--from the inside out, and outside in. Just the basics of eating were complicated. At every level, it seemed, I had to learn a different way of treating my body, and it was so unpredictable. It was good to not have to account for myself from day to day. To not have to worry about how I was affecting someone else's life. To not have to be concerned about trying to explain to another person how I felt--when it was so hard to do so to myself. With the right person, I supposed, interacting would be easy and nice. But it was hard to imagine anybody fitting into my life style.

Toward the end of August, a response to my request for money came from Mom and Dad. At first I was stunned. They were unable to help me financially. Dad had discovered that he had leukemia. They didn't know what to expect and were being careful with their money. They suggested that I ask Jack for help. I was deeply disappointed. Even though I understood, I couldn't help the hurt creeping in. *Look at the positive! All my anguish was for naught,* I told myself. *I am "saved" from living off my parents after all! I can be independent like Carol and others, juggling my piddling payments from month to month.* My ace in the hole was the shares Dad had given me two years before, devalued now, of course.

The only thing to do was to see this as my opportunity to really live creatively. To find the best route for me. I would learn that I *could* support myself, because that was the only choice. And I would do so without stress--because I would *choose* to. The news of no financial help was a big letdown, but it was also a relief. I reassured myself that much benefit would come out of it.

> *"To be fully functioning, then, we must be as welcoming of the new as we are comfortable with the old, as fearless of the unexpected as we are falsely secure in the planned."*
>
> *Leo Buscaglia,* ***Personhood***

That evening Jack phoned. It was nice to have him check in on me. Yet I had to bring up the financial situation. He was in no position to repay the money I had loaned him when we separated. He said, "You should have a plan and then you'll feel better."

And he'll feel better, I thought.

"You should think about your future."

I became immediately morose and nervous. How could I possibly think about and plan my future when every level of my life was changing from day to day? When I didn't yet have a handle on how strong or how mobile I might be once I started to heal?

What a joke it was to think of Dad suggesting that Jack could help me out financially or any other way. Jack had so vastly removed himself and written off any obligations he had toward me. Besides, ever since he opened his own architecture office, Jack had had a marked lack of income.

What *about* my future? Deciding or planning anything was impossible. It would have been extremely difficult to dive into househunting, selling, or moving right at that time. I didn't have the energy. I didn't know if I needed to locate a house without stairs or with a smaller garden and less upkeep. Yet, something had to be done to give Jack his share. I couldn't afford to buy him out, but I was determined that I would be able to someday.

I thought, *It would be so simple if I were a wife with a husband who has an income and who loves and could take care of me.* But, of course, that had never been the case and it was quite unlikely to ever happen. The challenge for me was to come up with some creative way to earn a living and to still keep my equilibrium. Thinking and speculating yielded nothing. I was so glad I would be seeing my counselor, Dr. Fleming, the next day. His listening and questions always helped me to clarify what I thought, felt, feared and desired.

When I saw Dr. Fleming the following afternoon, he said, "Don't take on the guilt and the burden that you brought on the illness. It's a neurological disease and it comes from many things. Of course, stresses may have contributed, but you didn't create the breakdown in the nerves. You didn't ask for MS ... It's not a good time to sell a house. Jack can wait because this is a special circumstance. ... Things will get better."

I knew that the key was unconditional surrender to WHATEVER --that I'd be led in the direction that I was supposed to be. I knew that somehow I was on a path that was for a purpose. I couldn't see it, but I was beginning to trust in it. I was still going to make a difference in the world. I was still going to contribute. "*How can I be right for somebody else, if I'm not right for me?*" asked the song. I was in the process of becoming right for me. That was what this challenge and this time were for. I wrote in my journal, *I accept this challenge and use this time and am patient with it and with myself. I need not be in a hurry to arrive at the end of my metamorphosis (if anyone ever does).* I continued writing, *Be patient. You don't need to rush on to the work, people and activities that lie ahead. They will be there soon enough in the right time.*

Right now, I needed to find out what worked for Barbara; to really know who Barbara was; to gain knowledge of her goals and priorities, desires, motivations and identity; to not be a clone of somebody else. Positive people could help, but it seemed clear that it was not a time to be emotionally involved.

> *"For all the sadness of closure, there is a new and joyful unfolding in the process of becoming."*
>
> *Mary Casey, from **Each Day a New Beginning***

It was discouraging to see my symptoms drag on and on. One night I felt stronger, so out I set on an evening walk. Little did I guess how quickly I'd run down. I found myself halfway around my neighborhood loop with no choice but to continue trudging on. Only a month before, such a short walk was an enjoyable stroll, and a year before it had been a nice jog. Now, in my tears, I counted the blocks, the houses, to my own house. Who would have thought it would ever seem so far away and take so much effort to reach?

With the coming of September, the days remained bright, but the sun was much less warm, less intense. The shadows grew longer earlier. Resting on the patio, I read my MS material, my healing books, and books loaned by my new friend, Sara. Sara had been referred to me to help out with the shop liquidation and had become a wonderful source of support--both in liquidating the shop and in friendship. She shared herself, her talents, her books and her experience with alcohol and drug recovery.

I particularly liked Sara's book of daily meditations, *Each Day a New Beginning.* The book was about "recovery." To my mind, we were all recovering in some form or another--from addictions, diseases, relationships, or limiting beliefs, fears, and patterns.

The phone kept me in the world. I talked to Sara and Ann regarding the shop; to Carol, to Peter, to my next-door neighbor, to the carpet cleaner. For the first time in years, I had the *time* to talk, and I had the desire. But I had to concentrate on calming down as I did so. For lightheadedness set in, and my arms got very weak holding up the phone. I continuously switched hands and I cradled the phone on my neck so as to rest my arms. Sometimes I'd just say, "Let me call you back. I can't hold up the receiver anymore."

Even though I continued to sit outside in the sun everyday, my tan was paling. The sun just wasn't as strong as it had once been. The light through my bedroom window each morning was full of shadows--no longer the stream of warmth bursting through, summoning me to hurry up and be in it. Colder, darker days were coming. I was determined to find joy and accomplishment and serenity in the fall and winter months.

But how I loved the patio when the flowers were bright. How cheery and healthy they were when they had not been beaten down by rain or cold. Golden marigolds mounded the beds and the purple and white of allysum rolled out from beneath the bigger plants. They burst with vigor, color and excitement. Yet all were in their places and there was a serene order about the garden space. In a matter of weeks, the maple, hawthorn and hazelnut leaves would be drifting over the beds. The cold would sap strength, and moisture would mildew and brown the flowers on their stems. The colors would fade and die and all would be shadows of green and brown and grey.

Remember, I told myself, *I can look forward to the crisp aliveness in the fall air.* No longer would I be compelled to be outside. There would be a comfort and a serenity in being indoors and warm. I could enjoy the cozy and comfortable surroundings I'd created in my house. *There will be days of books and music and rest. Friends will come and I'll share my warmth with them. The cats will cluster around the wood stove just as they clustered on the patio whenever I was there.*

All the while I will be resting and learning about my changed capacities and gathering strength. I'll continue to grow in my ability to meditate and to turn myself over to my higher power--to my guides within and without. I embrace the gift of this time--to learn, to grow, to seek inside, to discover myself, to establish my goals. What an opportunity!

> *"If I greet the day, glad to be alive, I will be gladdened by all the experiences in store for me. Each is making a necessary contribution to my wholeness."*
>
> *from,* **Each Day a New Beginning**

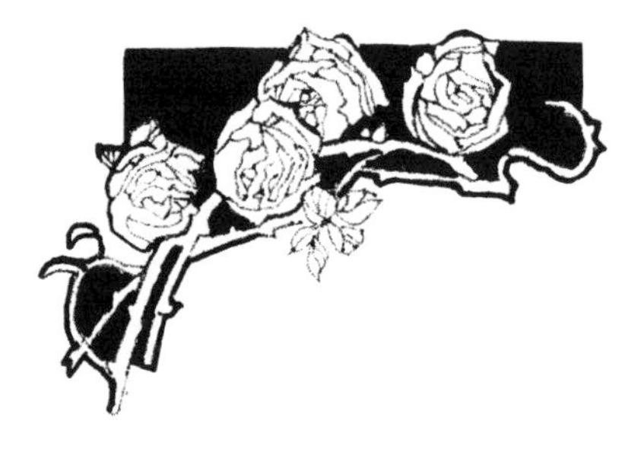

PART II

FIRST AWAKENING

Our first awakening reveals that our mind, conditioned as it is to superstition and tradition, is the prison-house in which we dwell.

Joel Goldsmith

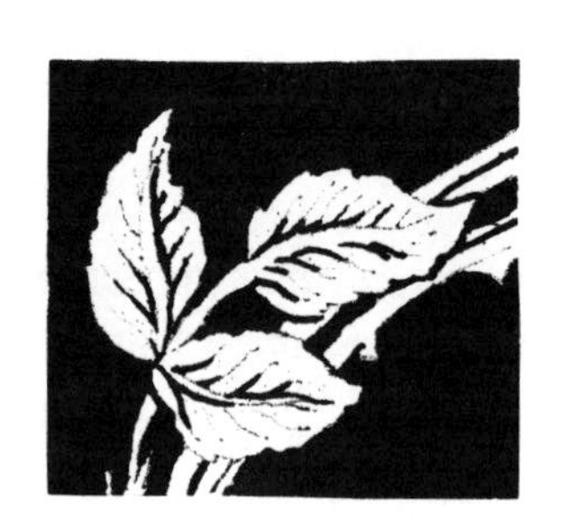

CHAPTER EIGHT

HAVING RECOGNIZED THE desirability of change, I didn't simply manifest it. The waking up process was fraught with delays and distractions and interspersed with triumphant milestones. I expected the hard work ahead would be alone. How wrong I was. I would soon discover a pattern of mine--that personal relationships are the arenas in which I work on my growth and changes and practice taking risks. Even as I embarked on those six months, anticipating solitude and the lack of interaction, a remarkable man appeared who became a teacher and a guide at the time when I was in need--as well as ready to change.

Jan Paul led me into myself as I sought to drop away the old. He probed gently and pointedly and was willing to call attention to my distractions, fragmentations and blindness. He supported and applauded my change. He reminded me about the quickly submerged goal of rest. His honesty mirrored mine as we both learned how to share love without attachment and obligation. With Jan Paul I learned how to celebrate my femininity and sexuality, to express my feelings and vulnerabilities, to accept and ask for help. Jan Paul's appearance on the scene was one of the first examples of my needs being met--before I could even anticipate them.

> *"Miracles are instantaneous, they cannot be summoned, but come of themselves, usually at unlikely moments and to those who least expect them."*
>
> *Katherine Ann Porter, from* ***Each Day a New Beginning***

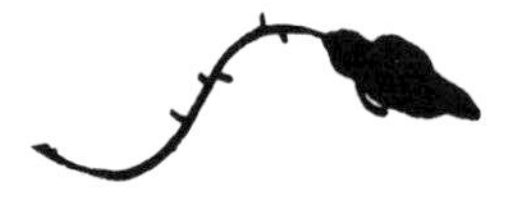

It was early Monday morning. After many lingering embraces at the front door, Jan Paul finally tore himself away and hurried off to work. I slowly wandered into my living room reviewing the incredible new twist in my fortunes. Within the space of two days, my cursory acquaintance with Jan Paul had taken a sudden turn toward a deeper involvement. I could hardly believe it. *Me! Intimately relating with Jan Paul Renner! Who would have ever thought it? Certainly not me.*

Jan Paul Renner was attractive, blond, and French. He was well-known locally as a vision therapist and seminar trainer. He was the kind of man--high-powered, stimulating, gentle--whom I'd always admired from afar, but never dreamed would be interested in me. Clearly, it was no mere accident that he had come into my life right at this point.

The time together with Jan Paul was a growing and a becoming, a contacting with myself, a connection with him, a pointing in the direction that I was going. He was interested in me and in my growth, but he was also careful not to push the teacher persona into our relationship. He had that very well in hand. He was committed to openness and eliminating games, unanswered questions, and self-defeating speculations.

Much as I thrilled to, and sponged up the closeness and the touching, the talking was what I loved. It was wonderful to interact with a man who made me think about what I was saying. He asked questions that required answers. When I proclaimed, "I'm going to love myself more," he asked, "How are you going to do that?"

With Jan Paul, right from the start, I was committed to behaving differently than I had in my relationships with Jack or with other partners. No matter how difficult or scary it might be, I was determined to express my thoughts and feelings. I had learned too well in the past how devastating had been my silence and hiding behind my mask of politeness.

The first evening with Jan Paul I felt clean and open and light as we covered some very difficult ground. We both wanted to be clear about how we would relate in the coming weeks. He understood my need for privacy and he needed his too. He wanted to feel free to phone, but didn't want me to perceive it as crowding. He wanted me to be free to phone him, but knew me well enough to expect that I might chicken out. We agreed to both phone and to both say exactly what was necessary and be honest about where we were or what we wanted. His courage in so caringly talking it out right at that moment made me especially respect and love him.

Originally I'd hesitated about getting involved sexually with Jan Paul. I had feared that if the sex turned out to be so-so, then the beautiful friendship we were developing would be doomed. I also entertained a limiting belief that I couldn't relate sexually to a man who was shorter than I was. Thank goodness I didn't let that belief stop me. Jan Paul was a wonderful lover. The sex, however delightful, though, was not the biggest attraction. It was more like a nice backdrop for all the other sharings. And, too, I was learning that I could create the kind of sexual encounter that I wanted. All I had to do was be honest. I could request, guide, and say "yes" or "no." It was up to me.

One afternoon, as he was readying to leave, Jan Paul said, "I just got that you are a very powerful woman. You've been weak and having insomnia because you're afraid of discovering your power. You're afraid of it because it is so powerful. It's the kind of power that impacts people. That kind of power is scary and that is why you find all these delaying maneuvers and mechanisms."

He gave me an affirmation to use: *I am a powerful woman overcoming my fears of being powerful.*

As of tonight, I told myself, *I'm powerful! I'm no longer a victim. I don't have MS! I have a weakness and I'm overcoming it! Power radiating! I unleash the power! I affirm it. I accept it! I encourage it! Everything is possible! My power is unfolding.*

After Jan Paul left, I sat in the living room with my furry companion, Betty, curled on my lap, and I thought about the implications of his words. When I had been my high-powered "self," I sensed that I intimidated others or was too aggressive and offensive. As I had become ill and weak, it occurred to me that now people might feel better about me, would not feel daunted or threatened if I could no longer be as I was.

I saw that what Jan Paul said was true. In some way, I had perceived myself as *too* powerful. But I didn't know how to handle it and at the same time relate to other people. So I shut it down and never allowed it to grow and develop. I supposed another term for "powerful" would be "honest." When I let myself be *me*, I overwhelmed and intimidated--because I demonstrated untempered, unguided power--immature. Now that I was physically weak, I had a wonderful way to prove that I was as humble, ordinary, and helpless as the next person. *What an incredible price to pay in order to gain approval!*

Later that evening Jack and I talked on the phone. When I talked about "power," Jack interpreted it as control over another instead of acting out of an inner resourcefulness, and he said, "Yes, you always intimidated me."

"What we wouldn't give to know
that it is okay
not to feel okay ...
... and to know
that it is okay to feel
powerful, magnificent, deserving--
even extraordinary."
Rusty Berkus, ***Appearances***

Surprisingly, despite my physical limitations, I was starting to enjoy the new texture of my life. For the first time in years, my days were unpressured by work and full of the sun and flowers outside. And, I was pursuing fascinating new avenues for growth--via books, records, tapes and classes.

I read *The Dow of Cooking* macrobiotically. Macrobiotics was a philosophy of eating local and seasonal foods while balancing root, round, stem, and leafy shapes and colors of vegetables. There were innumerable Japanese terms and ingredients that I was eager to learn about. I read Haiku, the succinct, Japanese poems, and listened, entranced, to my Sakura tape of haunting Japanese flute melodies. There was so much that I wanted to learn and absorb and to teach myself. At night, for my daily dose of humor, I watched MASH and WKRP. The hours raced by, and I couldn't possibly find the time in one day to attend to everything I was drawn to. *Where would I ever have found time to work in the midst of all this?!* I wondered. Best of all, I began to feel much more alert, clear-headed, and energetic. Finally, it became possible for me to absorb the information which I was encountering.

With Jan Paul, I could air the thoughts and fears that muddled my mind. One afternoon he led me through the "worst case scenario" of MS. I hated to think of it. Horrifying images assailed me--like that of Hawkins, the astrophysicist, in his wheelchair needing a translator to tell what he was saying because his vocal cords were so deteriorated. I saw myself having to give up my house and find one with no stairs. I imagined what it would be like to be helpless--dependent on others to drive me places or to feed me. I saw myself growing weak and fat and flabby in a wheelchair and never sweating again.

"The biggest fear you have," Jan Paul pointed out, "is that you will be incapable of looking after yourself, that you'll have to ask someone to do for you or help you."

So true. The paradox was that I had pushed so hard doing things myself, without asking for help, that I created exactly what I didn't want ... being so ill that I had to ask for help. That was certainly my lesson. That was the process. To find within myself the awareness and the courage to look after myself without pushing. I knew I had to learn to attend to *my* needs, not to act out of a requirement for others' approval or respect.

Jan Paul said, "It's such a gift for you to become aware of what your fears are. So many people never deal with their fears, and they go through life at the effect of them."

I saw things anew when Jan Paul pointed out, "You can say 'thank you' to your fears for the messages they give you. What a gift that your body becomes weak when you get racy or excited. Then you know that it's time to fall back, gather yourself, take a deep breath, slow down, get calm and then you'll be in a good place to carry on again."

He said, "You don't have to 'get rid of it' to win. You can choose how you react and you can be grateful for the gifts of the message--which remind you of who you are, what your priorities are, how you want to be functioning. 'Thank you, Weakness.'"

Thank you fears. You give me myself.

I found a passage in David Smith's book, *Healing Journey*, which I felt expressed what I was learning about fears. He was interviewing Juno, a 102-year-old Hunzakut man:

When I asked him whether there was any fear in Hunza, he laughed. There was fear everywhere. Fear was a friend. It comes "and gives us energy to climb, and to work, when we are in doubt."

Juno was saying, in effect, that fear was like the mountain itself--a friend if you embraced it but a deadly enemy if you were frightened of fear itself.

"It is not the conquest of fear that is important," he said, laughing again. "It is the putting of fear to work."

CHAPTER NINE

WHEN I PARTICIPATED in Jan Paul's vision seminar two years earlier and stopped using my glasses, I had been struck by his skills and talents as a teacher. At that time, though, I also perceived him as being insensitive and egotistical. The change in Jan Paul, obvious from the first day that he dropped back into my life, impressed me. In fact, it was one of the reasons why I was attracted to him. Somehow, something had made him turn around 180 degrees so that he had become incredibly sensitive and caring. He was aware of my inner needs and understood my tangled ways of tripping myself up. He was compassionate about that instead of impatient or belittling--which would only have served to antagonize me and make me defensive. Jan Paul said his changes were the result of his working with the Wings personal growth seminars, first as a participant and then as a trainer.

The seminars were held in Eugene and Portland. The more I learned about the Personal Effectiveness Seminar (PES) and the second level training, Cross Over, the more intrigued I became. But Jan Paul displayed remarkable wisdom whenever he talked about the things he learned from the seminars. He didn't push me to do them or even suggest that I should. At first.

It was an amazing time for me. I was discovering more and more that my thoughts determined how I felt. I was amazed at myself--at being able to *choose* to be so free and easy, so responsive, so affectionate, so accepting of the sex with Jan Paul. However, it wasn't being with *Jan Paul* that amazed me. The amazement was that I was having this sort of relationship with anyone at all. It was what I'd have dreamed of had I dared, and here it was, an unexpected miracle.

My body was amazing too. There were days when I was able to lie on my back or on my side and experience no tingling or weakness. *It's a healthy body!* I told myself. I could now move around the house more easily. Only sometimes were my arms, as well as my legs, a bit weak. I realized that a lot of what happened to me *did* come out of my head.

Sleeplessness was an example of how my brain misdirected my power. Insomnia had plagued me for years. So difficult was it for me to achieve sleep, that I hoarded my nighttime hours and my twin bed. I never asked Jan Paul to spend the night, fearing that I'd not sleep. Then one evening, Jan Paul pointed to the couch and said, "I'm going to sleep here tonight." We both settled in our separate beds around one in the morning. I didn't sleep at all. I read. I meditated. I visualized. I was so aware of his presence. I worried about being "up" and bright in the morning. I kept thinking that if I could talk to him I'd learn something. Finally, while I was meditating, I got a tremendous perception that that was why I'd stayed awake--to gain from him. So I woke him up.

He rose to the occasion beautifully--led me through my fears and worst scenarios, intuited some things, was alert and caring even at three a.m. He kept telling me "Thank your body ... You're so fucking powerful your body can get tight or loose just from thinking about something."

So I said, "Thank you, stomach, for the knots, for the messages. I'm no longer ignoring you. I'm regaining command. I'm attending to the excitement, stress and fears. Thank you for pointing them out--and you can go to sleep now because I'm handling it."

It was all fear--excitement--anticipation, living in the future instead of the here and now. I'd lay awake thinking, *I must sleep so that tomorrow I can be "up," alert, bright.* Thinking that if I didn't sleep then I'd perform badly. That I'd let people down. That if I was sleepy I'd miss out. The pressure to sleep was so intense that, of course, I wound up not sleeping. It was a terribly negative channeling of power.

On another day I realized another aspect of my power. It was especially rewarding because I discovered that, in fact, I could impact and empower Jan Paul. Up till then, I'd admired how skillfully he led me into myself, through dialogue and questions, gently pointing out certain things. I'd felt wonderfully cared for, felt his interest. Yet it seemed as if all I could give in return was my companionship and some healthy cookies.

Now, it was my turn to help Jan Paul, my chance to lead and guide and point out. We talked about his divorce and all that his wife was demanding. I began to sense that he was giving up much too much and not standing up for himself. As we worked it through, it did seem to be true and he began to get insights into his behavior and his fears. He went through a total mind shift and began to get very high and freed up.

I was flattered that he had shared so much of himself and that he had risked the vulnerabilities and fears by letting me in as he did. I was pleased that I could lend insight. And I was a little disappointed to discover that this man who I put on a pedestal was just like me. He also had garbage and fears and fell back.

In September, another opportunity came up where, in the context of the relationship with Jan Paul, I addressed old beliefs and patterns and opened to different choices of how I wanted to behave. Autumn Fest, in Portland's Old Town, was approaching. Tauni, Sara, and I planned to have a big sale. It was our last chance to unload the remaining inventory before closing the shop forever. Jan Paul offered to help, saying, "I'll be there to slow you down."

I was unsure whether Jan Paul would help or hinder, but I accepted his offer--and proceeded for the next week to carry around a backpack full of fears: *He'll be bored. He'll feel imposed upon. I'll be bossy. I'll get racy and pushy. I'll be like Anna, the lady who teaches the macrobiotic cooking classes, trying to carry on four projects at once and getting tighter and tighter. I'll get very weak and I won't be able to help, etc, etc.* The fears--I thought them and then they materialized.

I needn't have worried about Jan Paul. At the Autumn Fest sale he was just there--helpful, available, supporting me in taking breaks to rest. He lugged tons of stuff up from the shop basement, then sat outside and chatted with people and was very laid back. We split a beer--or rather, I had three sips--my first taste of alcohol in over six months! How great it tasted. I had only a slight, tight head reaction.

I could have been much more racy, but I kept it down. Even so,

I'd get into sales or conversations with people and wind up very excited and scurrying about.

"Are you resting?" Jan Paul frequently asked as we sat together or as I worked. Then he'd suggest, "Why don't you lie down for five minutes?" Once on my mattress on the basement floor, I'd realize how fast my blood was pulsating and how good it felt to lie there. Then I'd not want to get up again.

I stayed at the shop from noon till six o'clock and returned home still strong and relaxed. Wonderful! A phone call from my soft-spoken cousin Bob sparked a fresh piece of insight. As I hung up the receiver, Jan Paul commented, "I was watching the change in you when you started talking on the phone."

"What change?"

"You come from a real approval need."

Not wanting to acknowledge this, I said, "But I didn't even hear most of what Bob was saying."

"And why not? Why didn't you ask him to speak up? He knows you wear hearing aids."

I'd worn hearing aids for years. My hearing loss was one reason why I'd finally backed away from pursuing my love of languages. It took too much out of me, having to see the written word in order to make sense out of the sounds. Even with hearing aids and a telephone amplifier, however, I was accustomed to missing a lot of what people said, and I had mastered the art of improvising answers or inserting comments at what I guessed were the appropriate times -- a practice which had landed me in some hilarious situations. My experience had been that most people simply couldn't, or wouldn't, speak up or slow down their speech. Since it was a bloody nuisance to keep asking them to do so, I would most often just let it go. Because of Jan Paul's comment, though, I now looked at "hearing" in a different light.

I realized, *I didn't bother ... I didn't **choose** to hear Bob!*

And later, at the end of the evening, Jan Paul said, "Notice how your body is right now."

"Relaxed. Strong. Feels normal."

"How's your mind?"

"Relaxed, but stimulated."

"How was your mind in the shop today?"

"Stimulated/stimulated."

"When you've got your mind so it can be in this state--of relaxed/stimulated--all the time, you're going to be well, my friend."

I believed him.

"And you're going to be powerful. When you're like you are now, you're so powerful ... You have no idea how sensuous you are ... how stunning you are ... how powerful you are ... The greatest gift you have to offer is your calmness."

"Me?!"

"Yes. When you're like this how are you?"

"Relaxed."

"And when you're relaxed how are you?"

"I'm more open."

"And what else?"

"I listen."

When I can listen I can heal myself. I will be able to take care of myself. I can give ...

All those years I had been so busy doing. So busy choosing not to hear and not to listen. So I paid no attention to my own needs and therefore very little attention to the needs of others. Now the body was taking its own way of grabbing my attention. In a crescendo of pain and weakness I heard all that was going on inside of me, all that I had been ignoring. All that I had chosen not to hear. I was listening now.

I told myself, *When I've learned how to listen to myself and to the voice within me, I will also be able to listen to others ... My greatest gift ... I'm in the process now of evolving to that place.*

"How do I arrive at that relaxed state?" I asked Jan Paul.

"You'll find the mechanism. That's what this process is all about. One tool ... slow down your talking."

"The change of one simple behavior can affect other behaviors and thus change many things."

Jean Baer, from ***Each Day a New Beginning***

CHAPTER TEN

SEVERAL WEEKS HAD passed since I'd seen my old friend and lover, Peter. One afternoon he came over. I was too weak to sit up, so we lay on the bed talking and sharing. I said everything that I needed to and wanted to. All honesty. I no longer feared bringing up subjects that I once avoided because they might be too touchy, too direct. I didn't fret about how he'd respond or fear that he would reject me. I told myself, *If he does, he does. If he can't handle discussing his wife, his girl friend, sex, his feelings for me, then that's his problem and responsibility, not mine.*

I told Peter about Jan Paul and how I perceived that even the sex was an important part of the unfolding of my own power. I felt that I was learning from my involvement with Jan Paul how to transcend my fears of relating sexually to him and to others; that I was starting to overcome my inhibitions about asking men what they wanted and my fears of truly allowing myself to shine out; I was beginning to release my apprehensions of expressing my own desires and needs; and I was opening up to allowing all the passion and power to flood out of me without reservation, without putting on the brakes.

I had changed so much, I told Peter, that I was now committed to total honesty in sex, to feeling free enough to tell a man what gave me pleasure, and to asking him what gave him pleasure. I was learning that:

> *"Love is a school, and sex is a very important part of the curriculum. What do you learn in the school of love? You learn to be more loving."*
>
> *William Ashoka Ross, Ph.D.,* ***Sex***

That night as Jan Paul and I made love, I wanted to give him pleasure and he encouraged me to talk to him. I'd never before done that to a man, even though I'd always responded so well when Jan Paul talked to me. With an effort, I let go of my inhibitions and just tried any words that came. I wasn't polished, but it wasn't that difficult. The talking helped to excite Jan Paul and he had a raging climax, which left me feeling pretty wonderful, knowing that I'd been instrumental in creating that. I'd finally felt as if I'd given to him as much pleasure as he was giving me.

The following evening Jack stopped by. We talked about Jan Paul and about lovemaking. I couldn't keep back my overflow of good feelings about the relationship with Jan Paul and told Jack, "Jan Paul is a super lover."

Lifting his eyebrows, Jack asked, "What does he do?"

"He's very giving and very sexy."

Talking about it later with Jan Paul, he laughed and related to Jack's comment. He said, "Men are always interested in more doing. It's the content, not the doing. It's where the man is coming from when he does these things. I've 'done' the same things to my wife or other lovers, but if I'm coming from an ungiving place, then there might be zero response."

A week later Jan Paul and I were talking about our past sexual experiences. He told me about one girlfriend, how they both had climaxed together, and how she'd had three orgasms aside from that. He asked me, "How do you feel when I tell you about such things?"

I could honestly say, "It pleases me that you feel so free in our relationship that you can tell me about it. I'm also pleased that you've had the experience of her and of good lovemaking."

I didn't tell him, however, that I immediately started comparing. *Can I have simultaneous orgasms with him? Can I have three orgasms? Will he want to make love to me if I don't?*

In bed later, my mind was racing, even though I knew it was ridiculous to compare. How could I equate my experience with another woman's? I kept looking for the flip side, for the positives ... *I'm capable of **five** orgasms!* or, *This is a chance to genuinely accept my own experience--no matter what that might be.* At the same time, I felt pressured and feared not having an orgasm at all.

In the end, I was able let it be okay to have *my* sexual experience, rather than striving to emulate someone else's. Once I relaxed and let go of the pressure of comparing, the sex was very good--and different. It was the most silent time we'd spent together. But it was nice and sensual and I had three orgasms.

"To change one's life:
Start immediately
Do it flamboyantly
No exceptions (no excuses)."
William James

I gradually took my changed behavior into the arena of family relations. It was late September, the day before my parents were to depart on a trip to China. I felt an urgent desire to communicate my love to them before they left the country. Yet I feared I'd seem silly, seem too expressive taking the risk of saying, "I love you." But I wanted to do it. The question was how? I decided to meditate on it. I sat quietly for a few moments. Inwardly, I sensed: *Phone--trust that I'll say whatever is right.*

That's just what I did. It was one of the best conversations I'd ever had with my mother. Twice I told her I loved her and Dad. I told Mom about Jan Paul. She said, "He sounds intelligent," and immediately switched the conversation to asking about Jack. Personal subjects like men, romance, divorce, emotions, were subjects my mother preferred to avoid, so the rest of the phone call remained safe and superficial. She told me how she'd enjoyed reading the book I'd sent--Shirley MacLaine's *Dancing In The Light*, about how we create our own reality, and said she was thrilled with the corsage I'd sent as a bon voyage gift.

I was very glad that I called. It was a risk because I feared being vulnerable, feared that my parents would not acknowledge my outreach. It was an emotional stretch for me, an exercise in self-expression to the two people who I considered my most critical audience. It was one more opportunity to pull myself upward--and how satisfying the results were.

"You may never know which choice was "right" but you can always tell which you'll respect yourself for making."
*Read and Rusk, **I Want to Change, But I Don't Know How***

CHAPTER ELEVEN

WHENEVER I TOLD people that I had MS, I felt divided within myself. To say the words outright seemed a reinforcement of my identity as an MS victim. I also felt split because, inwardly, even as I spoke, I *knew* that this was going to change ... that I'd overturn it. But I couldn't *not* tell people. It seemed important for others to know what I was up against.

Perhaps I perceived that my future achievements would be especially noteworthy if I were classed as a survivor, an overcomer. People would look at me and say, "She did that--and she did it with MS!" or "She did that, in spite of her handicap," and "She BEAT MS! What a person!"

Why would I have set up such a program? Ever since I was little, I had admired survivors and had devoured books like *The Diary of Anne Frank* and *Mawson's Will.* Always wondering how *I* would behave and if I would persevere in a critical situation. Always thinking, "How terrible--what so-and-so endured. Could I do that?" Always hoping that I'd never have to go through any horrible experience in order to find out. Yet it seemed I needed, indeed, to find out--to affirm for myself that, in fact, I could and would and did survive. That I would be recognized as a survivor in spite of my desire to avoid the act of discovering that identity.

> *"Out of every crisis comes the chance to be reborn, to reconceive ourselves as individuals, to choose the kind of change that will help us to grow and to fulfill ourselves more completely."*
> *Nina O'Neill, from* ***Each Day a New Beginning***

I continued reading books on healing and change and about people who had transcended their difficulties. These inspired and reassured me as I took baby steps toward trying new behaviors and to understanding what was happening with my life. One such book was *Joy's Way* by Dr. Brugh Joy. It spoke so powerfully to me that I felt overwhelmed. My mind was boggled as I turned each page and found clear and penetrating expressions of the same ideas that I was discovering for myself.

Joy was explaining exactly where I was. He experienced his own disease as a signal from a major force within him that demanded change. The choice, he said, was either to follow the outer mind or to follow the soul. Like Joy, I had vacillated over the choice for months. I saw the illusions of the stability, as well as the roots, that I had created with Jack and with my flower shop. I thought that I could maintain what I'd built, and at the same time expand into my inner consciousness and come into contact with my true path--that I could do both at the same time.

Like Joy, I had rationalized all the positions I'd taken in my life. But all along, there had been a sense that there was a deeper pattern and path, and I ignored it. I felt that Joy was right, that my refusal to look at the path had been part of the cause of my disease.

As he explained it, a disease could put a person on a terminating course which was transformation--either to physical death, or toward a transformation on a living side. If any transformation was to be effective, the patient had to change his attitudes and life patterning as completely as he would if he were dying. There could be no half measures and no compromising. Sweeping changes were required and each one of us alone knew what those changes were. I was in what he called the "challenge" state--where I had to marshal the courage and the clarity to make the necessary changes.

There were countless pages to which I related and that were so profound that I could only quickly clutch at them and then move on, returning later to try to grasp them in a deeper, more lasting way. I felt so dumb. Why couldn't I read and comprehend and then be able to explain it to Jan Paul or Carol or Jack? What I was learning was so important--the necessity of letting the outer mind drop away and letting the soul's true course flow. Yet, I feared I couldn't convey this realization to others.

I was impatient, too. I wanted to leap immediately into the

experience of deep meditation and the inner teacher and trusting my inner voice. I felt incredibly immature in my level of awareness and my ability to conceive of higher states, let alone achieve them. I wanted to dash out and locate a group to meditate with. I wanted to find a teacher to guide me. I wanted to put in hours of study, reading, writing, meditation.

I could only trust the process. I told myself, *I am at the beginning of the journey and I still have to shed the old baggage that I've been carrying for a long time. If I hurry forward before I have organized my body and my spirit for the next stage, I will not be prepared. The journey will be too difficult to understand and will be meaningless and chaotic.*

I drew inspiration from Virginia Satir's words:

> *"I want to get you excited about who you are, what you are, what you have, and what can still be for you. I want to inspire you to see that you can go far beyond where you are right now."*
>
> *from,* ***Each Day a New Beginning***

One day as I was talking to Jan Paul about my impatience, he said, "You are pursuing your transformation in the same way you've gone about work or projects."

As usual, he was right. I was still caught in the old web of being achievement-oriented. I didn't feel that I was getting any further along in my healing or my wholeness unless I'd read X many books or listened to certain tapes or meditated X times or conducted my visualization three times a day. No wonder I didn't get to bed until midnight. Endless items had to be checked off before I could consider that I'd made enough progress on my journey. I was driven to get there--to achieve my state of equilibrium and power and control over my stress. What a contradictory statement!

"I want to move on," I complained. "I'll live my life so much better when I get to the next phase of the journey. I want to hurry forward and fulfill my potential and to step into my power *now.*"

"You are missing the point," said Jan Paul. "The point of the journey is to learn to accept the place where you are. Wherever you are is necessary and important for your particular path. It has pertinence and is to be savored, enjoyed and explored."

But I didn't like hearing that. I compared myself with others--with the Wings trainers, with my friend and mentor, Katherine, in Australia, with Jan Paul, Brugh Joy, Frances Horn--and I stewed impatiently. I was all too aware of Brugh Joy's statement: *"This time lag space is where a lot of people drop by the wayside. They've started their program, but don't see their true progress."*

> *"Longing for a different time, a distant place, a new situation, breeds discontent. It prevents us from the thrill, the gifts offered in this present moment. But they are there."*
>
> *from,* ***Each Day a New Beginning***

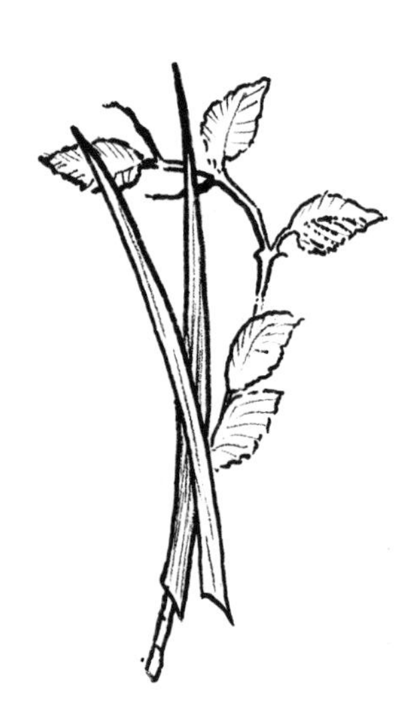

CHAPTER TWELVE

AT LONG LAST, in mid October I attended one of the Wings introductory evenings. It was designed to offer a sample of what the five day PES (Personal Effectiveness Seminar) would be like. Jan Paul and an attractive older woman were the speakers. He looked very elegant, handsome and poised with his tailored, fawn-colored suit, blond hair and blue eyes. I enjoyed watching him and listening to his fluid words with their lilting French accent. All the while, I related his comments to the audience to what I knew of him personally and privately. I was proud of his intelligence and articulation and of being a friend to such a fine man.

I liked the presentation and felt that I could definitely grow into deeper levels of resourcefulness and effectiveness if I did the PES seminar. At one point in the evening, we sat in small groups and did a process, saying to each person, "My experience of you is ... " It was totally intuitive and quite incredible. The insights that people picked up simply from sitting across from one another were amazing. Usually we are so caught up in the experience of what someone says--"I'm a lawyer, a wife, 42 ... " In this process we cut right through these superficial definitions of each other to the heart of who each one of us was.

I'd wondered what people would say about me. They picked up on the same things that psychics and Jan Paul had. "You're hard to get to know. You keep yourself aloof and apart. Underneath you're warm and soft. You want to please other people. You're nervous. You have a lighter side and can be fun." Pretty incredible. They *had* me, and all I did was sit in the circle with them. So different from the time I did the est trainings, when I was told, "Wipe that smile off your face, Barbara," and I felt silly and chastised for being who I was. Here, I didn't feel put down for being myself. I simply gained personal insight and realized that what I saw was what also came across to other people.

After that night, Jan Paul and I frequently discussed my doing the Wings seminars. He was eager for me to take the PES training, knowing it would make a big change in my life. "But," he would add, "it scares me too."

"Why?"

"Because I'm afraid I'll lose you."

He said it many times. I guessed that he feared that once I became personally effective, I wouldn't need him so much. Perhaps he thought I'd be so powerful that I'd go flying off to perform great wondrous works elsewhere. To my mind, it seemed that I'd be an even better partner for him once I became stronger within myself.

The issue was not with me, so much as it was with Jan Paul. "Every time I talk about losing you," he said, "it lessens the fear. It's old stuff coming up. The lesson for me is to be able to encourage and allow you to grow and not let my old negatives and expectations overwhelm me ... to allow whatever happens to happen. We can be friends, even if we do not stay lovers."

It was from the Wings people that I first heard the statement: WHATEVER I RESIST I GET. That certainly described me. I resisted not sleeping and I got that. I resisted disease and I got that, too. *Stop resisting. Start experiencing*, I told myself. *Each experience is happening to me right where I am in my current state of beingness. Each experience is a learning process and a growing one and is exactly the experience I should be in at that particular moment.*

Jan Paul often stopped me in mid-sentence or in mid-activity to ask, "How do you feel right now?" In order to answer, I would have to get in touch with my feelings and only then would I realize that I felt strong or weak or peaceful or up-tight and I hadn't even noticed it.

He would also say, "Did you hear what you just said?" or "Listen to what you said." My words were such a metaphor for the way I had programmed myself. For example, I talked to one lady about making her wedding flowers and, as I talked, I realized I didn't want to do it at all. "I got tired," I told Jan Paul. Negative things made me tired. For years I had repeatedly said, "This flower business is a pain in the butt," and look what I had--exactly that!

> *"When people make changes in their lives in a certain area, they may start by changing the way they talk about that subject, how they act about it, their attitude toward it, or an underlying decision concerning it ..."*
>
> *Jan Illsley Clark, from* ***Each Day a New Beginning***

I knew I needed a break from all my transformation focus. I also felt that it was important to continually put myself into fresh situations, especially those in which I could practice the art of relaxing or learning to tune in to my inner self. In late October, my friend, Carol, and I drove east to the Cascade Mountains and participated in the women's music workshop at Breitenbush Hot Springs.

On the second morning at Breitenbush, I lay naked, luxuriating like a lazy lioness on a warm granite slab that sloped into the laughing river. To my right, silvery grasses painted lacy patterns against a cobalt sky. Around me ringed the fiery trees of autumn, blazing against the forest green. Insects hovered like fluffs of lint. Here and there, hot springs spewed lazy drifts of steam. Women's voices chimed across the silence and occasional snatches of melodies floated heavenward while the bubbling river chanted a chorus.

How expansive a space of non-doingness can be, I reflected. *Who would have ever dreamed that I'd sit in the sun and compose a song, let alone two?* I was opening up to new creative processes as I opened myself to new behavior. I was learning how to sit on a rock in the sun and simply be. I was learning from the trees and the sun and the river. *I am discovering that other things happen when I simply lie back and think or don't think, see or not see, hear or not hear*. I was learning what it was like to sit without a book or tapes or letters to write. Instead of bringing paraphernalia and activities into nature, I brought only an unplanned, open mind and body. I realized, *As I am, I become, grow, expand, create, open and awaken.*

> *"Through spontaneity we are reformed into ourselves. Freed from handed-down frames of reference, spontaneity becomes the moment of personal freedom when we are faced with a reality, explore it, and act accordingly."*
>
> *Viola Spolin, from* ***Each Day a New Beginning***

Back in Portland the following Saturday, I attended another Wings "sampler" workshop. It turned out to be a triumph in several ways.

About 80 people gathered at the Red Lion Inn to participate in the all-day event. It provided a preview of what we would encounter in the PES (Personal Effectiveness Seminar). We were directed in several experiential processes which were particularly aimed at working through the layers of feelings we had toward people. I discovered that I couldn't identify feelings, that I felt only confusion, that I could only say to Jack, (my process partner who represented him) "I can't express myself to you. I feel as if you don't understand me or what I'm saying. I feel as if you only hear from your point of view and you twist around what I say." I told "Jack," "I realize that doesn't make you bad or immoral or me that way. It just makes it impossible to feel as if I'm really communicating my point of view to you."

I discovered that I had squelched my real feelings so completely, for so long, that I was quite out of touch with how I felt. I had made a virtue of avoiding confrontation or drama in my relations with Jack--and he with me. We both had no idea that there were deep feelings of resentment, anger, disappointment and being put upon.

I had always been so careful to be fair. To see both sides and to keep up the polite facade. The irony was that my behavior still came across to Jack as being hard-shelled, closed off, angry, judgmental, resentful. All the things I buried and wouldn't express overtly, because they weren't "nice" or "fair to Jack," still managed to be expressed in covert, subtle ways that I wasn't aware of. In the day's processes, I recognized this.

I wondered, *What do I do now with that knowledge*? Was it worth it to express all these things to Jack at such a late stage? I supposed so, since it would be a way to complete the cycle of the relationship. But I decided not to dredge up the old negatives with Jack. Thanks to the day's workshop, I had a better understanding of how we'd confused one another, but now I wanted to focus, instead, on where we were. We had managed to come so far in being able to be caring and honest with each other now that we were no longer living together.

I didn't realize it then, but the pattern of avoiding feelings and conflict played a critical role in my health issues. Yet, it would be another three years before I would sufficiently address this pattern--with amazing results.

At the end of the day's activities, there was a dance, and in a visible way, I got to see that I really was making progress with my health. After my body first crashed, whenever I wanted to imprint a vision of health and wholeness on my being, I would visualize myself dancing--alone or with a partner. I equated being well with being able to dance. All at once, without fanfare or notice, my image came true. I didn't dance a lot, but I *did* dance. I was aware of the great leap forward that the dancing represented. It seemed strange that the moment had come about so naturally and simply, that it didn't seem out of the ordinary.

While at the dance I was also pleased to notice how far I'd evolved from past days of desperate dance floors. I felt good about myself and was unconcerned about having to connect with dancing partners. I fell into immediate rapport with one gentle, heavy-set man with whom I danced and talked throughout the evening. I enjoyed our chatting, but I was also aware of the gaps in the conversation, of the spots where I'd throw in a phrase or a comment simply to fill the empty spaces and to keep the bridge of words propped up.

I remembered many other such situations from school and travels. I certainly had come a long way from the bright, charming, conversational coed wanting only to please and to be asked to dance--to not be left out. Here I was, still bright, perhaps charming, yet more real, more completely a woman in touch with herself, still wanting to please and to be asked to dance, but there was no more waiting and watching in covert, silent desperation.

It was late when I got home, exhausted from my long and intense day. All I wanted to do was sink into a delicious sleep. Just then the phone rang. It was Jack. He said, "I wonder if I can come over."

"I'm tired and in bed."

"Oh."

"What is it?"

"Nothing that can't wait."

"If it's important, come on over."

"I can come another time."

"I don't want you to feel that I'm rejecting you. Is it something that came up today and you want to talk about it?"

"I wouldn't bother you for something trivial."

"I don't want to let you down."

"It wouldn't be the first time ... I don't want to screw up your evening."

I got him to come over. My tummy clenched tight. I thought, "Oh, boy, he's going to go into the stuff about the divorce, about Jan Paul, or money or the house. That's all I need."

My tightness was from my fear of blowing it. But then I realized that I never really do blow it. Here was a chance to choose to come to Jack from my own power and integrity and from my heart. I didn't have to allow *his* projection to chip away at my integrity.

When he started talking and it was about how to deal with his latest lady and her Christianity complex, I relaxed as if I'd just been spared a firing squad. After a couple of hours of my questioning, leading and suggesting, Jack said, "Thanks, Tweet. I hadn't thought before of you as someone I'd get answers from, but I feel like I have." He added, "You guided me very well. You'd be good at it. You're really becoming an insightful person. I couldn't talk to you this way before, but now that we're not involved I can."

I was touched by these comments coming from Jack.

He continued, "I admire you ... for the person you're becoming ... for the way you're dealing with your problems and with other people's problems."

I told him, "I have a sense that I'm going through this now in order to learn and grow and that I'm in a process and someday I'll share from this experience."

He said, "I believe you are. I admire your intellect. You've not had to use your intellect for a long time and you let it go. Now I can see it sharpening."

"Thank you for sharing that," I responded. "You know, though, it's not the intellect so much as it is being willing, at last, to listen and follow my intuition. My 'skills' are the result of mimicking the way Jan Paul talks with me."

It seemed unnecessary to bring up the things I learned in the Wings workshop. Individually, and together, Jack and I had each grown and come so far. As Jack left I felt a surge of tenderness. "I love you," I said, reaching up to give him a big hug.

"Oh, Tweet, you're a very special person."

Wow! I thought. *Jack speaking in this way! How that helps to verify my sense of the rightness of what I'm doing and of the direction I'm going.*

CHAPTER THIRTEEN

I WAS DETERMINED to maintain my body's muscle tone and circulation. Ever since the MS diagnosis, I had been attending a therapy swim session at a nearby pool. Three times a week I joined a group of forty or so men and women at the shallow end of an extra-warm, Olympic-sized, indoor pool. There were people with all kinds of disabilities--some extremely crippled. I met three women with MS, two of them very incapacitated--stooped and shaky with feet that were thick and purple from lack of circulation. The pool experience made an impact on me which took me a while to absorb and understand.

I was fascinated watching the casual way these people got around. Slipping mincingly out of their wheelchairs on to the floor next to the pool and then sliding slowly into the water ... working out doggedly around the pool with someone helping them, or supported by empty plastic gallon bottles, generally keeping up a chatter of conversation both in and out of the pool. They swung out of their chairs onto the toilet, or wheeled themselves under the shower--and it was so natural, simply a way of life.

I was impressed by the spirit, but I didn't know if I identified with them. On the one hand, I said to myself, *That will never be me*, or, *I'm strong and will stay that way*. Then I'd catch myself walking more gingerly, almost as though being with these crippled walkers gave me permission to be less robust, less sure-footed. Then I'd think, *I must **not** identify in this way. I will walk as surely and as purposefully as I feel within. Can I not give them more if **they*** *identify with* **me**, *if they see a member of their group walking strongly and surely? They know that I have MS. Perhaps my example of health will somehow be positive for them.*

I didn't know how or in what way it would happen, but I felt that there was some long-range reason why I was experiencing the time with those withered, tottering, yet spirited people. I felt that I had something to give them. The nagging question was; *Do I have to become just as weak and crippled in order to contribute?* The answer was emphatically *NO*. I realized that I could never contribute effectively or significantly from a place of weakness. I could and would contribute from a place of strength. The lessons from those days of physical weakness were helping mold the inner strength that I needed. Paradoxically, once I had developed my inner strength, I simultaneously and subsequently generated my outer strength.

This truth was evident three years later when my ability to give blossomed in circumstances which brought me in touch with several older people. Chief among them were my dying father and my crippled mother. Instead of fearing or judging their incapacities, I was able to relate to and identify with their frustrations. I could offer myself in a patient, understanding way that I doubt would have been possible without my own experience of illness.

At the therapy swim I met Rosemary, a bright, slim red-haired woman with MS. She told me about her church and invited me to one of the prayer meetings to receive a laying on of hands. I'd heard of such things and eagerly looked forward to learning what was involved. And, just maybe, it would even help.

On a cold Wednesday morning in late October, I met Rosemary at the Holy Trinity Church. It was a Catholic parish, and I thought, *This is pretty far-out stuff for me.* After the prayers and singing, a large, jolly woman, Martha, came over and said, "Rosemary said you might be willing to have a laying on of hands." I responded, "Sure. I'd love to. I don't know anything about it, but would like to have the experience."

Martha said, "There's nothing that you have to do. Just sit there and let it happen." She explained, "Sometimes people feel warm, like a furnace, or they may feel nothing. We may be moved to place our hands in different spots, or we may be moved to say words that probably won't make any sense to us, but they will to you."

Two women knelt in front of me with their hands on my legs.

Rosemary was to the right and the grey-suited, grey-haired Martha stood by my right shoulder. A young woman, Barbara Jo, completed the group with her hands on my left side. I felt a lot of warmth from their hands and I also felt extremely peaceful, rather unusual for me, since I usually knot up in the stomach when I really want to "get" something.

Martha put her hands over my ears and my hearing aids whistled. She asked if I had pain in my right abdomen--I shook my head, "no"--and put her hand there. As the women were finishing, Martha repeated several times, "You're lovable just as you are. You're lovable just as you are. You don't have to change." She didn't know why, she told me later, but that was what she was impelled to say.

Afterward, the black woman said, "I kept hearing, 'I'll show you. I'll show you,' over and over."

The comments of both women seemed well suited for me. I was the person who wanted to be transformed and changed and who also felt unlovable. I was the one who was searching for answers to my way of being, who wanted some spiritual direction, and through it all, I felt so uncertain.

Barbara Jo said, "I get that you're worried about God. Don't worry about the *form* of God. Whether it's Christian or Buddhist or whatever. Just let God show himself to you in whatever way he comes."

I didn't appreciate her wisdom at the time. Only later, did I begin to follow her advice and cease looking for God in different forms.

> *"Invisible is he to mortal eyes, beyond thought and beyond change. Know that he is, and cease from sorrow."*
>
> ***Bhagavad Gita**, 2:25*

At home that night, with the fire leaping cozily in the wood stove, I sat down to take a trip into another world, the distant, nearly forgotten world of my past. As part of my process of self-exploration, I reviewed my old journal notebooks. How strange it was to view experiences with past people and events as seen from the context of who and where I now was. I could see the old patterns, the ones that I was currently so conscious of needing to change. As a young woman I had written about wanting to fit in, wanting approval of others--and all the while I knew that what mattered was my own. Yet here I was 16 years later still learning that lesson.

I had written of the changed considerations that arise as soon as one becomes involved with others. How did one determine where the line was drawn between consideration and constriction? I had concluded that when I had to consider how others would be affected by my actions I was no longer acting out of my own totality, from my own heart's singular purpose.

I read on. I saw that my behavior with men was affected by their possessiveness and their jealousy. On the *Canberra* sailing to Australia, I hadn't known how to communicate to my Aussie suitor that I enjoyed his company and wanted to be his friend, but I also wanted to be allowed to be complete in my own self. As a result, he and I both spent the voyage in taut confusion. Reading my journals afforded me a revealing measurement of how far I'd progressed since that time. I now recognized the need for honesty in communication. Still, the difficulty came in bringing it about.

In the old hitchhiking days, I'd had choices: comfort and security versus the unknown. I remembered the lonely New Zealand salesman who paid for hotels and meals and who detoured to show me special sights. He would have continued doing so indefinitely, asking for nothing more than a kindly uncle type of companionship. But we really had nothing in common, and I felt stifled. After several days together, I realized that I couldn't continue sacrificing myself for the easy ride and security. Choosing the unknown, I asked him to leave me at a youth hostel.

My later diaries showed how the disintegration with Jack had started as early as two years after our marriage. The disillusionment, boredom and lack of spark settled in so quickly. How could I have failed to recognize that that sort of stagnation was utterly wrong for me? I turned outside of the relationship for stimulation--to the garden, food preserving, books on nutrition, the flower business, to racquetball, to myriad projects. I filled myself up with activities because I was unfulfilled in the marriage. There was so little excitement or spark between us.

How valuable it was to look back in time. It reminded me of how things had once been, and thus helped me to acknowledge that, indeed, progress *was* being made. It reinforced the importance of persevering. Seeing the mistakes of my past helped me to recognize that I *could* change the future. I was not in bondage to yesterday.

> *"To look backward for a while is to refresh the eye, to restore it, and to render it the more fit for its prime function of looking forward."*
>
> *Margaret Fairless Barber, from* **Each Day a New Beginning**

CHAPTER FOURTEEN

NOVEMBER BEGAN COLD, raw and depressing. I discovered yet another body disharmony. One bleak day I lay in bed with Jan Paul, tears dampening my face. I couldn't get away from the thought, *What next! Candida--fibrousitis--MS--and now herpes!* It seemed that I was breaking down one piece at a time. That I had to attend to so many facets of my body. That I went from restriction to restriction. No sugar or fruits or carbohydrates. No fat. Special diets. Restricted movement. Now there was all this attention on my vulva, rinsing and drying it and applying cream all day long.

Both Jan Paul and I had been dismayed at the discovery of herpes since neither of us had ever had it. When I asked my gynecologist how this could be, he explained that the virus could have remained latent in my body for 20 years, and that when a person has a weakened immune system it's not unusual to see infections like herpes become evident. I grew sad as I saw how far down I'd driven my body. *Be thankful I'm as well as I am!* I told myself. Herpes, after all, was hardly a problem compared to the many other diseases I could have had. I was able to at least be grateful that it wasn't in my eyes, as it was with my cousin, Evelyn. I couldn't help noticing, however, the irony of herpes cropping up just then when I genuinely wanted to be sexually active. It would have been a great excuse to use with past partners when I didn't want to have sex.

"Our immune system is only as strong
as the dosage of self-love, self-acceptance, and self-care
that we administer to ourselves daily."
*Rusty Berkus, **Appearances***

The next day I hit rock bottom. Reading the Help Wanted section of the paper did it. I had no burning desire to do any of the listed jobs and the ones that might be interesting required all kinds of credentials and experience. I wasn't afraid to go out and acquire the necessary credits. My problem was that I had no passionate commitment to any one thing.

I'd recently written down what I considered to be my "burning desire." It was to interact with people. To have many, varied, interesting and deep life experiences. To stimulate people and provoke self-awareness, growth, and healing by virtue of my own enthusiasm, experience and expression. Nothing I read about in the newspaper sparked my interest or lured me to the point of wanting to focus on it alone or to making whatever sacrifices might be necessary.

In the afternoon Jan Paul came over and brought his sex book. I felt quiet and withdrawn. We went into the bedroom and, as we were making love, I felt the vast difference between his aliveness and my deadness. He was so vital and interested in arousing me and in being together. I could only simulate involvement. My thoughts were dwelling on how much of a struggle the whole process of life seemed to be and had always been for me. Eileen Caddy said, on her tape, that life was not meant to be a burden. Yet all I could see was the battling and the continual struggling.

I thought how ridiculous it was to be in a life where I had to do verbal exercises in front of a mirror in order to be positive. How futile all the effort was in the long run. How burdensome just the act of getting to sleep had become for me. How exhausted I was all the time. I took pills to sleep and then I was tired all day because of the pills. If I didn't take them, then I was fatigued because I didn't sleep. The pills created constipation and so I had to take more pills to deal with that.

I was weary of having to be so exclusive with my body--of having to take hundreds of supplements, of having to eat select foods, of having to affirm my health and love for myself every day, of having to work so hard at simply being able to function. Just looking ahead to doing my Christmas cards--something that should have been fun--weighed like a huge boulder.

As Jan Paul made love to me, I was thinking of the sleeping pills in the bathroom cabinet and how simple and restful it would be to just take them all and go into a deep sleep. I'd never again have to deal with all this struggling. I couldn't keep back the tears. Sadness came welling up from some deep, bottomless place within me. I responded to the lovemaking, but my thoughts were all on death. There was a certain sly delight in knowing that I could be so intimately involved with a person and yet retain the complete privacy of my thoughts. No matter what Jan Paul and I were doing, I still had a private, secret space that he couldn't begin to fathom existed.

I kept my face turned away. Even so, eventually Jan Paul realized that I was very quiet and not participating as usual. *How can I possibly talk to him?* I wondered. *He'll think me melodramatic and negative and tell me to do the PES training.*

So I didn't talk. Crying silently, I kept thinking about how beneficial my death would be to the few people around me. It would settle the house for Jack and his future would open up with money and without encumbrances. I would leave my clothes and my share of the house equity to my friend, Carol, and that would be a real windfall for her. I'd leave my journals to her, too, and maybe she'd do something with them where I hadn't.

Mom and Dad would be off the hook as far as having to concern themselves about me. My sister would inherit half the property instead of only a third. Just getting out of all the obligations and worries and fears seemed utterly attractive.

There were really only two reasons why I hesitated. One was that I was terribly curious to know what would happen if I didn't die. The other was that I believed that I was given these lessons to be learned in the course of all my lives. If I didn't handle them at one point, I'd just have to handle them later in another life. Not that I wouldn't have minded taking a break for a while. I thought it would be wonderful to perhaps be with other spirits and to get my batteries recharged.

I finally did talk to Jan Paul. He was very good, of course. Supportive. Loving. Cheery, even.

> *"[People] attempt to live cautiously in the safety of established patterns. They do not feel fulfilled, yet they have found a formula not of success, (whatever that is), but of avoiding failure. This is a living death ..."*
>
> *Read and Rusk,* ***I Want to Change, But I Don't Know How***

CHAPTER FIFTEEN

SOME INTERESTING IDEAS and a new form of guidance came my way via a series of tapes by Napoleon Hill, the author of *Think and Grow Rich.* Mr. Hill talked about his system of guides, which made wonderful sense to me. He had a guide for each of the important areas of his life, and he relied on them to help him handle things.

I started trying out this new concept. It felt so right to say, "I don't know what I should do about Christmas--or whatever. I'll let Edward (my guide to Peace of Mind and Decisions) handle it." By giving that part of my subconscious a personality, it was easy to visualize myself literally handing over a condition or question to that "person." Then my conscious mind let go, breathed more freely and I knew that the issue was being handled.

There was the day when I was nervous about asking my singing teacher to let me sing with Carol at an upcoming recital. Since I had been away from the lessons for so long, I feared and expected rejection. I sent Barnhill (my roving ambassador) ahead to clear the way. By the time my teacher and I talked, she'd already spoken to Carol and all was agreed to.

Another day I was nervous about phoning a lawyer to ask for a discounted half hour of his time. I projected that he'd agree--and he did. The appointment was made for the very next day. I didn't worry though. I trusted that I'd be prepared because I turned all the details over to Orvill (guide to Overall Wisdom). When I sat down that night to prepare the details for the meeting they just flowed out.

I'd hemmed and hawed about travelling to California for Christmas and, finally, I left the decision up to Edward. The next day, without further vacillation, I simply made my calls and arranged a flight. I was wait-listed for better travel dates. Instead of fretting about the dates, however, I just left it all up to Barnhill.

Giving my guides names helped me to characterize them. Hippocrates was in charge of health. Uncle Will handled my Financial Prosperity. Edward, of course, was in charge of Peace of Mind. Hope encouraged me that I could be and do things that I dreamed and conceived of, and Faith gave me faith in my ability to achieve them.

Blossom was my guide to opening to the love that I could give and which was waiting for me when I opened myself up to it. Rose guided me to opening the romantic, poetic side of myself and to eliciting it in others. Pop was the guide to Patience. I always thought of Pop, my grandfather, so patiently kneeling before his flower beds --lively riots of color which his blind eyes couldn't even see. Still he nurtured and coaxed those flowers day by day.

Orvill was my guide to Overall Wisdom. His purpose was to guide me in how to derive benefit from the experiences that came to me. He showed me how every experience, positive or negative, was grist for my mill. He helped me to learn from my experiences and guided me so that I wouldn't repeat the same mistakes over and over. I had a special guide for humor and that was Uncle Charlie. Barnhill, as my roving ambassador, handled such matters as clearing away the parking spots when I drove downtown and making room for me on the wait list at the airline.

With the guides in command, I no longer needed to fear or worry that I wouldn't ask the right questions or that I'd say the wrong things. I simply handed those anxieties over to my guides and I trusted that all would be handled.

It's been a long time since I've used those imaginary guides. But looking back, I recognize the value of that concept. For it was a stepping stone to the inevitable leap, that of handing ALL over to the inner WHATEVER. It was a way of learning how to put something out of my worrisome mind, and to trust that some part of me would handle it.

When I met with Mr. Benson, the lawyer, I spelled out my house proposal along the lines to which Jan Paul had guided me. I had finally decided that I *would* ask Jack for support. The support payments, however, would be canceled because I would buy Jack out of the house. When Mr. Benson pointed out that, in essence, I was asking for the house and that all Jack and I would be doing was exchanging $11,000, I was bowled over. In a flash, I recognized what I was asking--for Jack to just give me the house. I couldn't relate to such an idea, and I knew Jack would explode over it.

Suddenly I saw how making a proposal of that nature was literally throwing down the gauntlet. I didn't want to battle Jack, and I especially didn't want him to think he had lost me as a friend. Surely such a proposal was not something a friend would initiate. What could I do? I realized I must turn inside for answers, that there must be a way to ease my own burden without depriving Jack of the benefits to which he was entitled. I couldn't cheat him out of the house by asking for an amount of support.

I asked myself, *Does Jack owe me support?* No. Just because society chose to give the man that role and obligation didn't mean that it applied to us. It wasn't Jack's fault that I was ill (or was it?). If he had been the sick one, I'd not have felt obliged toward him and I'd certainly have resented it if he had tried to make me support him in a post-marriage arrangement. In reality we each had chosen to have no more obligations toward each other. It seemed downright underhanded for me to present him with a proposal that would wipe out any proceeds he'd otherwise get from the house.

I want to act out of love. I told myself. *Asking for support is acting out of fear and selfishness*. All my reading was telling me that when we act from love it comes back to us again and again. I needed to try out that concept. And, I *wanted* to pay Jack his share. There was nothing to be gained by cheating him simply because I happened to get ill right at that time. I asked myself, *Why should we go through a lot of confusion only to finally arrive at this resolution anyway? Are we big enough people to come straight to this point?* I decided I could give up the idea of support, if he could give up immediately receiving his share of the house money. That seemed fair to me. I hoped it would seem so to him.

"Make the rules of your life such that even if the worst imaginable results come from your efforts, you will still love yourself."

Read and Rusk, ***I Want to Change, But I Don't Know How***

CHAPTER SIXTEEN

IT WAS THE end of the first week in December. With a sigh of satisfaction, I finally sat down in the living room surrounded by my furry companions. Each cat occupied itself in its own particular way. Gherkin was totally zonked out on the floor, beyond awakening, even though the wood stove crackled only inches from his white fur. Betty was perched, half-mellow, half-prissy, on the couch behind my left shoulder. Wooster had finally curled into a furry urchin on the couch next to my lap after completing an ever-so-cautious reconnaissance of the velvet cloth underneath the Christmas tree.

As I sat listening to Gregorian chants, I savored the memories of the evening. Carol had come with her son, Jesse, and Jan Paul had brought his daughter, Beatrice. We all set about decorating the tree, popping popcorn and drinking mulled cider.

Jan Paul and Carol visited while Beatrice, a real live wire, and I decorated most of the tree. Jesse, being older, was much more casual and mostly interested in keeping the popcorn in supply. I was pleasantly surprised to find that instead of hoarding the tree trimming for myself as was my usual custom, I actually enjoyed sharing the activity with others. I wasn't anxious because ornaments might not be hung where I'd prefer to put them. It was *fun* to share the activity, to have the laughter, the chatter and the confusion. In the end, the tree looked smashing. It hardly mattered at all where the ornaments were placed.

So I sat, long into the night, enjoying the colored lights and the festive conglomeration of animals, shiny balls, popcorn and mini marshmallow strings. I drank in the peace and the orderliness of the house. For once, the tables were cleared, the counters bare, and the books and papers put away. I'd tried something new--sharing my tree and festivities--and it had been a wonderful success.

Two days later I canceled my upcoming Christmas flight to Santa Cruz. It wasn't hard to do. I'd originally eliminated my mental seesawing by making the reservation. Now it was easy to just decide not to use it. Again, no flipping and flopping. I honestly didn't feel up to the travel and the preparation it involved. Going to Santa Cruz meant a whole week of juggling my special foods as well being busy cooking and planning with Mom.

I also felt extremely reluctant to spend the money. The reality of my economic situation was sinking in. I had $600 left to cover the December and January bills and then only $1,000 left in savings. That was it! Funny. That looked so drastic. Yet I believed that something would come in before I used my last dollar. *Where from?* I continually asked.

My father had hinted that he might sell the pasture land which he had deeded to us three children several years earlier. Although such a transaction would inevitably result in the destruction of his peaceful, rural neighborhood, I couldn't help hoping that he would negotiate the sale. It seemed like it would be the perfect solution to my financial problems. But there was no way of knowing whether or not the sale would really happen.

A few days later, my life and my finances took on a new dimension, one that I wasn't sure I wanted. Suddenly I found myself employed by someone else--for the first time in over 12 years. Ruth at Charmant, the lingerie shop which I had once provided with flower arrangements, eagerly accepted my offer to help out over Christmas. "I'll commit for three months," I said. "If other jobs I've applied for come up, I reserve the right to take them." Although I had mixed feelings about working, it felt good to know that I would have *some* kind of income.

The first day at my new job set the tone for what I could expect in the coming weeks. The long stretches of standing tired my legs. Whenever possible I sat down, but that meant retiring into the storeroom where the tiny step stool was kept. The other ladies were nice and the place was lovely and welcoming and efficiently run by Ruth. My duties were minimal--in keeping with my minimal wages.

I found myself divided within. On the one hand, it was pleasant to let the time wade slowly by as I chatted with the two girls or looked at the lovely lingerie. Simultaneously however, I simmered, bored with having no more than one task to accomplish. My sole purpose was to sell the lingerie, but when no customers were there I felt the need to be doing something. *Can I stick it out for three months?* I asked myself over and over. I wondered if the tiny income was worth the upheaval in my time. I could have been using those hours to read, study, write, to be with myself or with friends.

At home, Jan Paul asked, "What's the motive?"

The motive was to make money. But I wondered if 20 hours a month at $4.25 an hour was sufficient for the time, travel, gas, parking and bus tickets.

"It's more of a validation that you're employable than for the money," said Jan Paul.

On my next working day at Charmant, I at least enjoyed the first hour. I tried on all the 34B bras, learning about their makes and cuts and discovering that there actually was a value to be found in a $40 bra. I began to see this lingerie experience as one more piece of my growth--of my personal awareness. I was in the process of learning to love my body and of learning to love the men in my life. Part of that learning was sexual and related to all aspects of sharing my body with another person. Until that time, I'd been hesitant to carry this learning into dressing in a sexually enhancing fashion. *This association with lingerie will help open that door,* I told myself. *I will see to it that it does.*

While at Charmant, I would listen to the men who came in to buy. I would observe the women who bought with men in mind. I'd have a chance to become familiar with beautiful underwear and to get a sense of it being an everyday item--something that I, too, could want for myself. I would try on garments and develop a more casual, natural attitude about wearing such things in front of a man.

"Choosing to live life sensuously refreshes you and opens you to the ongoing mysteries of life. That's why sensuousness can be the beginning of spirituality. Sensuousness leads you from your restless random obsessive thoughts back to your skin, to your flesh, to your senses which are your interface with the world. And spirituality? Spirituality leads you to your center."

William Ashoka Ross, Ph.D., ***Sex***

One day, after leaving Charmant, I stepped into some strange territory in regard to my relationship with money. I treated myself and the world as if I had all the wealth I needed. I treated my money as an abundant gift that I had available to share with those around me. All the while I was thinking of Napoleon Hill's statements about getting back ten times what you put out. I also thought of how I'd functioned with a close-fisted money mentality and I'd not attracted money to me. I'd certainly not felt abundant. I decided that day to pay people for their worth, just as I would if I really had money.

I paid my hair dresser extra for spending extra time on my hair. I simply shared a Christmas concert ticket with Rosemary and didn't worry about the cost. I told myself, *It's time to share my abundance and start acting as if I have enough money to pay people and give to people as I feel I want to.*

I bought pots of flowers and placed them about the living room, bright, cheery red poinsettias. Repeatedly I told myself, *I deserve to live in beauty and to bring beauty to myself and to the people who will be coming to my house. I am* ***not*** *frivolous. I* ***do*** *live in abundance. My survival* ***is*** *assured. There is* ***no*** *guilt. I* ***can*** *have flowers in my life!*

Without realizing it, I'd begun to access a universal principle: that abundance, as an attribute of God, is infinite. I was beginning to perceive that I lacked abundance in my life in the degree that I believed it was finite. Even a millionaire can live in misery, believing he doesn't have enough. Although this principle is taught by most religions, my only "proof" of its truth is the example of my own life. As, in ever greater degrees, I've ceased clinging to money, possessions, and even to places, experiences, and people, and come to view myself as a funnel through which these infinitely available attributes flow, I find that I experience an incredible abundance of them.

> *"The most powerful thing you can do to change the world is to change your own beliefs about the nature of life, people, reality, to something more positive ... and begin to act accordingly."*
>
> *Shakti Gawain*

Another incident invited me to scrutinize myself and my beliefs about abundance. Eleanor, a woman whom I'd met through my singing lessons, invited me to a ladies' luncheon at her exclusive club. I was delighted to have the chance to step out of my daily grind of focusing on healing and changing. I met Eleanor at her house before the luncheon. When I stepped into the sumptuous setting in which she lived, I was amazed that anyone could live that way without the pressure of working. I decided that Eleanor must have struck it rich when she divorced her husband, but I also realized that there was no reason why I couldn't also have the elegant house and clothes and the freedom to have fun and to travel.

All I have to do is to continue to change my thinking, as I am now doing, I told myself. Seeing myself with all the abundance I needed was such an about-face from the way I'd envisioned myself for so many years. I'd hobnobbed with poor people for so long. It was nice to think of interacting with people I liked and who were also well off. I was beginning to see that it was no longer necessary for me to wear my poverty like a badge of virtue and seek approval because I was just scraping by.

> *[on passing an elegant "expensive" restaurant] " ... partly we were kept out because of our stupidity and narrowness. We had never in our lives dined in so elegant a place and had not enough intelligence or imagination to see ourselves doing so. And we were satisfied with the little world we knew. Proud of it even. We had no desire to increase our experience. It never occurred to us to ask about prices instead of deciding, without knowledge, that they must be beyond us. It never occurred to us to look inside to see if, actually, we would like to eat there. We accepted the legend both of the desirability and the unattainability. When either or both might have been false."*
>
> *Jessamyn West, **To See the Dream***

The weekend came when I worked my first eight hour stretch at Charmant. I watched the clock all day--something I'd not done for years. The best part of the grindingly slow day was my 45-minute lunch break, which I took in the women's bathroom across the street at the library. I ate in the warmth of the antiseptic tiles and read the Hazelden Center's book, *Each Day a New Beginning.*

What a treasure that book was. It keyed in on all my reasons and experiences, my motives, processes and hopes. I asked myself, *What is this Charmant experience teaching me*? Somehow, I knew it had to be exactly what was right for me at that time in my life. *It is teaching me humility and patience. It is teaching me that I must be creative if I am to find work that is satisfying. I'm learning that I absolutely do not want to be a shop clerk, that I do not do well in a laid-back, non-demanding setting of mindlessly working for someone else.*

There were more eight-hour days at Charmant. How many times did I watch my watch? At least I made progress with Helga, the "German General." I was at last getting some softer words, some smiles from her. How anybody could spend a year there--straightening the bra and panty cubbyholes and organizing and reorganizing the racks of day wear. Helga was obviously intelligent. She just was not very ambitious.

My anxieties about not having enough money and not having an identity kept pushing me back into old habits. One particular night was an excellent example of how I kept ignoring my body's demands and my inner messages. It was a freezing 21 degrees outside. The directions to the fat lady's apartment were terrible. I had to trudge all over her icy apartment complex with my bulky box of ribbons and bags of supplies. As I taught the seven (mostly overweight) women how to make bows, I wondered again why I got myself into such situations. I became extremely tired and bored. I lacked enthusiasm and couldn't muster the energy to put out that extra effort to help the slower women better grasp the principles. The evening dragged beyond ten o'clock, as I knew it would. When I finally got home, the heater was not working.

Accepting the invitation to do the bow making party and pushing myself to do the other activities of the day had been contrary to what my body was telling me it wanted. I wanted to rest, but I persisted with pushing and doing. And I knew that I could expect the ensuing days to be more of the same. I felt out of control.

"People who stay in miserable situations, sacrificing their self-respect, their needs unsatisfied for fear of losing what semblance of a relationship or security they have ... are saying: I'm afraid to take the chance: my self-respect isn't worth the hassle."

Read and Rusk, ***I Want to Change, But I Don't Know How***

CHAPTER SEVENTEEN

DECEMBER FOURTEENTH, MY 40th birthday, was a memorable and special day. At six o'clock I met Carol at the Inner City Hot tubs. We were the only ones there until first Ellen, and then Mark and Anna, arrived. We managed to all crowd into the same tub and the same sauna and I loved the chatting and sharing as we sat and soaked and sweated.

After an hour, we evacuated the tubs and went over to Old Wives Tales for dinner. It was such a lovely group of people--a real mixed bag. Jack came and I was pleased. Marilyn, too, from the past. Sara and Don from the flower business present. Carol and Linda from the friendship and music part of my life. Mark and Anna from the macrobiotic side. Pam from a workshop, and Ellen from a chance meeting last April.

Beforehand, I was anxious. Who was I to ask people to interrupt their busy holiday schedules to spend time celebrating my birthday?! The audacity of it startled me. Then I wondered, given that they came, would they enjoy each other? Would it be awkward and would I feel responsible for everyone sitting there wondering why they had come?

Silly borrower of worries. Each person took care of his or her self and made their own point to converse with those nearby. I sat myself right in the middle where I could hear the best and was able to yo-yo between Mark and Sara, Jack, Pam and Anna.

When the evening was over, I gathered up my gifts and paid my check. Walking out to the parking lot with Carol, I felt wonderfully high and bubbling with delight in the evening. It had gone off well. Everybody seemed to enjoy sharing and meeting. I was full to overflowing with the love of them all and with their friendship for me.

Leaving the party and coming home alone felt good. I never considered what it would have been like to have been a partner in the evening with a man that I loved. I didn't even miss Jan Paul, gone to Eugene. I felt happily content to come home and practice my guitar strums for ten minutes, sing a song or two at the piano and then sit down beside my brightly lit tree. Betty lay curled up next to me. I felt exquisitely complete.

As I tackled the issues each day brought, it was so hard to know whether or not I was making the right decisions. I had choices about how to take care of myself, but how was I to tell when I crossed the line from being self-nurturing to being self-harming? I could only try out what felt right at the time, as I did when I attended a Christmas concert with a couple, Tom and Diane. They had invited me to join them afterward at a mutual friend's house for a dinner. Originally I'd accepted, but as I sat through the music, I decided to act on my real feelings, which were that I thought I'd get more value out of just going home and being quiet. I worried that by turning down the invitation I was allowing myself to slip into a hibernating mentality and that somehow I'd miss something that I'd regret later. Yet how silly. If I wasn't there, then I couldn't have missed anything. At the concert, I had a sense of the forced conversation with Tom and Diane. I realized, *I'm learning to kiss goodbye those people and activities from which I no longer grow.*

I told myself, *I must begin living as if I'm already 80.* I'd always thought that when I was 80 I would be wise and eccentric and free enough to behave as I desired--that somehow having lived that long I'd command enough respect to be able to carry it off. But I was beginning to realize that that was a false image. I asked myself, *Why should I wait another 40 years in order to say and do and be as I want to be? Why must I deny my true self right now simply because I've not crossed a certain arbitrary age barrier?*

> *"[Self-actualizing] people are capable of behaving in what seems to be the most extreme forms of "selfishness"--they protect their time, say "no" to unrewarding social invitations, recoil--naturally and without much guilt--from toxic people, situations, jobs and responsibilities ... they know what they must do with their time and energy and then determine to do only that."*
>
> *Marsha Sinetar,* ***Do What You Love, The Money Will Follow***

On Christmas Day, I had to again determine what was the best path for me. I knew Jan Paul wanted to spend time with me that evening. He'd phoned first thing Christmas morning, crying and wanting to be held, propped up. There was lots going on with his divorce and with his wife. I found it difficult to understand how she could scream and rage. How could anybody be that way to someone they've lived with? I felt a bit miffed that Jan Paul was crying and phoning me. Yet he had always been available for me to do the same, and I certainly had taken advantage of that accessibility. I realized that this process with Jan Paul was teaching me to allow a man to have the same weaknesses and tears that I did. *Why, after all, should I expect him to "be a man" any more so than I am?*

The day itself was delightfully laid-back. Jan Paul and his sister came for an afternoon dinner. He and Elizabeth arrived at noon. We prepared food as we visited for two or three hours. Finally it was ready and we sat down to our healthy macrobiotic Christmas feast. Both Jan Paul and I appreciated the food. We felt wonderfully virtuous eating a special meal which was wholesome and healthy as well as tasty. I think it was the first festive dinner I ever experienced when I felt really good afterwards. Instead of feeling leaden and ill with too much rich food, I felt energetic, light and well satisfied.

After Christmas dinner, I tentatively told Jan Paul that after the full day, I wanted some time to myself, and I was relieved when he readily accepted that. I was so grateful for a relationship in which we could be that way. How good I felt being true to my own need for solitude and privacy. It would have been so easy to be caught in a trap of thinking that I needed to be with people. I took my time with Jan Paul and other people and relished it. And I took my time alone and felt comfortable with that.

There were occasions, however, when I told Jan Paul that I needed to be alone and he whined and cried. Then I found myself pulling away. I knew that he acted this way out of love for me. Yet it also seemed like need. At those times, he seemed to interpret my choosing myself as rejecting him. But I didn't think it was. I realized that I had two choices of people to be with. One was with Jan Paul, or other friends. The other was being with Barbara. For 40 years, I'd spent very little real time with Barbara. Now I was choosing to do so.

I enjoyed getting acquainted with the many unrealized facets of Barbara's personality. I thrilled to the unfamiliar feeling of what it was like to love and accept her. I wanted to be with Barbara just as I wanted to be with Jan Paul--for the enjoyment of her spirit, for the revelations of who she was, what she thought and desired, where she was going. In the 13 years with Jack, there had rarely been those quality times with Barbara alone. Now I longed for it. I savored it. And I could not berate myself for choosing it.

> *"Natural **self-ishness** is cutting the bullshit. It's centering your life in you, mastering the art of looking after the person who is you. And not unless you excel at selfishness can you truly give."*
>
> *Read and Rusk, **I Want to Change, But I Don't Know How***

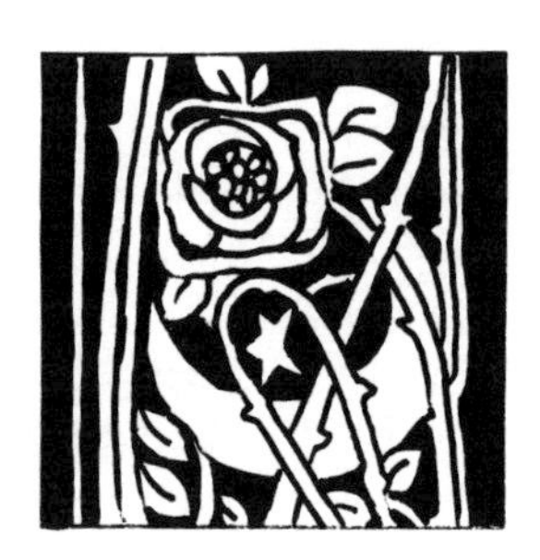

CHAPTER EIGHTEEN

THE END OF the year was approaching, and once more I re-read my old journals. I began to see my travel journals of long ago as a log of external experiences which paralleled the expanding interior awareness of the young woman named Barbara. As she had negotiated her outward journey, so too, the inner person had felt, perceived, developed, feared and triumphed.

I rediscovered the girl who had written in her journals in Monterey in 1967. I was amazed at her expression and articulation, at her perception in regard to her parents, at her descriptions of train rides and beaches, fears and doubts. Who would have ever dreamed that that same girl would be a 40-year-old woman in Portland, Oregon? That she'd sit typing by the fire on a winter night, content in her aloneness, stimulated by her typing, and surrounded by the woolly, lumpy bodies of three flaked-out cats?

How would that girl in Monterey have possibly anticipated the years of struggle and doubts and the beautiful 40th year's blossoming? That 21-year-old girl expressed herself artfully. The 40-year-old woman was cumbersome and slow. She was, after all, out of practice. She was not mentally tuned up as that girl had been from years of stimulating and scholarly environments. The words, the descriptions, the adjectives, did not come rolling naturally onto the paper as they once did.

So there was much delight in discovering the expression and the somehow surprising maturity of that younger woman. I also discovered her intolerance and her impatience toward her mother. It wasn't a conscious cruelty, but it must have hurt nonetheless. How could that girl have guessed that the day would come when she would come to know compassion and show great caring for her mother and even share some special, almost intimate moments? How satisfying it was to read and to know that the hurts that were once inflicted were exorcised, that the girl and the mother and the father really did come to a time of loving and openly enjoying each other.

On New Year's eve, as the hour approached midnight, I sat in the warm living room. My white terry cloth robe was colorfully splashed by the lights of my Christmas tree. The three cats were sprawled around me on chairs and rugs. With mixed feelings I reviewed the year. In some ways it had been such a struggle. Then I remembered 1983 and how difficult that was. 1984 had given me similar struggles, but somehow they weren't as frightening as they had been in '83. Looking back at both years, I could say, "I survived." Not only did I survive, but I grew. That was the difference between 1983 and 1984. Much of my suffering and anguish sprouted from the same circumstances and fears. Yet it wasn't until 1984 that I acted, that I made changes.

I viewed the year ahead with hope--because it was new--that I would hit on the right combinations of spiritual, mental and physical disciplines that would make my body well again. Then there was the flip side--the fear that no matter what I did there would not be a change, or that the changes would be negative. I managed to maintain equilibrium and positivism as long as I discerned that I was making progress. Then days would come along, like the last few, when my legs ached and shook, and then in crept the insidious doubts.

Physically, I supposed that my condition was no worse than it had been a year before. When I considered that it wasn't until August of 1984 that I started consciously altering my behavior, I realized that I should be grateful for my progress. Indeed, it seemed that I was holding the line. It was reasonable to expect that 40 years of spiritual and mental negativity and physical abuse would, after all, take some time to exorcise. So the experience was one of patience. Just as working at Charmant was. Just as trying to find "the" life work was. Evidently I hadn't yet learned the lesson of patience, despite its being taught on several fronts.

One thing I was coming to realize was that it was *acceptable* for people to have periods in life when they had no job title to define themselves. How easily we all slipped under the umbrella of occupational definitions. I, of all people, should have known how real and vital I was when I was in a mode of being neither one title or another. How readily I'd forgotten that I lived that way for years when I was overseas. At that time I had identified myself as a Traveller. Hence I had some purpose in knocking about various places in the world without being a this, that, or the other.

Just as before, I told myself, *I am again a Traveller, but not to distant geographical places. I am embarked on an inward journey of discovery that is taking me to exotic realms of the mind and spirit. Just as those travel years were not a time for structure, so is this a structureless season.* But, despite understanding this, I continued to define myself as the owner of Bloomers even though the shop was gone, and I still worked (to my detriment) on wedding flowers in my garage to maintain that structure.

Accept and acknowledge that it is okay to be in limbo. Moving from one career to another didn't mean that one day you worked at one job and the next day you walked into another. This was a Big Transition Time. How could I possibly be certain what steps I wanted to take? Nobody could expect that. It *was* acceptable to rest, read, write, meditate, gather information and attend seminars, all the while not necessarily having an answer to the question "What do you do for a living?"

The movement is the important thing and I can only do it at ***my*** *pace.* Hadn't *something* looked after me wonderfully well to this point? What had been the use of all my worrying about money? What would be the use of worrying about it from this point on? If there was one lesson I could take to heart it was that I *was* looked after. *Why not accept that and drop away all the old habits of worrying?*

The Garden of the New Year

"The echoes of last year, its sorrow and laughter,
Have died away.
The song-voice of the New Year
--encouraging, hope-imparting--
Is chanting: "Refashion life ideally!"

Abandon the weeds of old worries.
From the forsaken garden of the past
Garner only seeds of joys and achievements,
Hopes, good actions and thoughts, all noble desires.

Sow in the fresh soil of each new day
Those valiant seeds; water and tend them
Until your life is fragrant
With rare flowering qualities ..."

Paramhansa Yogananda

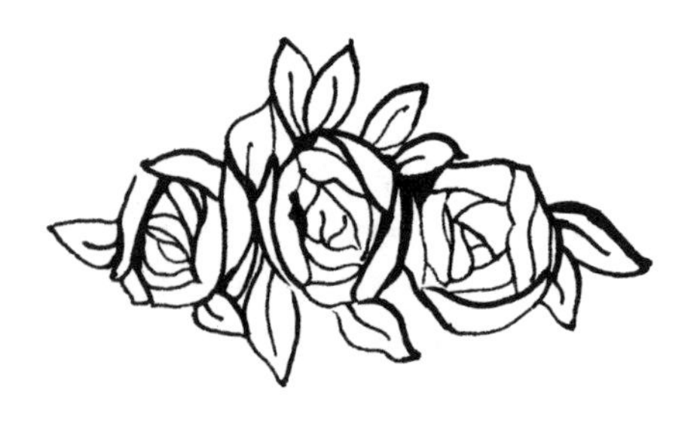

PART III

AWAKEN YOUR HABIT-DULLED SPIRIT

The New Year whispers:
"Awaken your habit-dulled spirit
To zestful new effort ..."
Paramahansa Yogananda

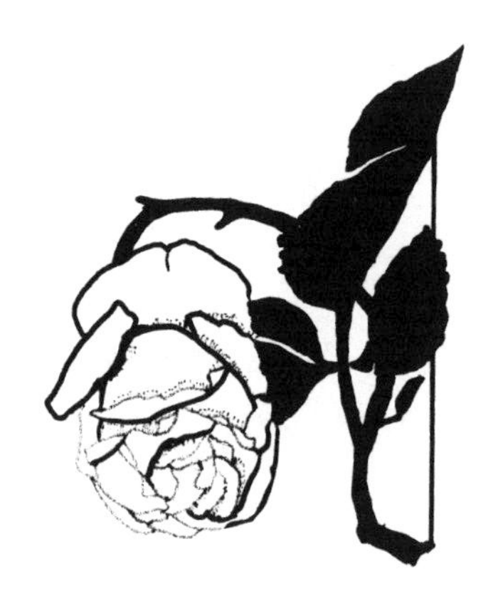

CHAPTER NINETEEN

IT SEEMED THAT everything I did took me farther away from the quiet serenity of periods alone, of healing time. I continued to buy books and they piled up unread. I was too rushed to meditate, too busy to swim or walk, too hungry to fully prepare a meal, too pressured to take a moment to be with my friends. Where had I heard all that before?

The long days at Charmant left me sapped. I couldn't get excited about checking, tagging and folding bras and panties and I especially loathed the limp pure silk bras that seemed to be all straps and which were impossible to fold in a neat manner.

After each session at Charmant I straggled home from my bus stop and lay down exhausted. I didn't want to, but sometimes I became emotional and self-pitying. I felt such a longing to rest, to be able to sit or lie down during the day as the need arose. I longed to take an hour for exercise. I asked myself, *How can I do any of that without someone to take care of me?* I felt so much the need of that someone. But, of course, I knew that I must access that care for myself.

I felt trapped by the schedule which kept me from the pool. I was frustrated when I looked at my body and I saw the doughiness, the bloated stomach, the flabby legs, the saggy face, the puffy baggy eyes, the double chin, the tiny, shrunken breasts.

Love my body, I told myself over and over. *Love it for its rejuvenating. Love it for looking as good as it does. Accept that this is a temporary condition. The exercise will come again. The muscles will tone again. All in the perfect time.*

Most of the pressure arose from my fears of being unable to survive financially. The situation at Charmant was making it clear that I had to look at work from a new perspective. I cast about for ways to make money. I read, made lists, interviewed and phoned people. I had procrastinated for several months about installing a renter in the lower level of my house. Now I set the wheels in motion. I hired Jack to remodel the downstairs so that in addition to it's own entry and bathroom it also had a self-contained kitchen.

My money supply was getting tighter and each credit card had been used to its limit. I sent away an application for yet another Visa--I who had never owned one until four months before. I didn't know how else to survive. I planned to use the Visas and then when --and if--Dad sold the Santa Cruz property I'd pay off everything. I'd buy Jack out of the house, pay doctors, taxes, and credit cards, and maybe I'd even have enough left to support my going back to school if I decided that was what I should do.

One morning, after a restless night, I awoke early. My stomach churned nervously. I was aware of the magnitude of the decision that was evolving. There was no doubt that it was the right decision, yet I hesitated, delayed and resisted it. I had to get out of Charmant, where I was withering on the vine. Every time I went in, I felt as if I lost a little more of my essence. Yet I couldn't stop thinking about the paltry sum of money that waited for me if I kept going. But I also thought of each Saturday from January until April and I couldn't abide the thought of spending eight long hours stagnating with bras and panties and price tags, especially if I had to share them with Helga, the "German General."

I had been developing an interest in going back to school and studying to become an occupational therapist. It seemed like an interesting and viable occupation for me. Excitedly, I rang Jan Paul and told him what I was thinking of doing. Instead of being pleased for me, he got hurt and pissed. I just said, "Call me back later when you feel like talking," and hung up.

He called back, thanking me for letting him be in his own stuff. Walking together later in the afternoon, it was good to be with him. He said, "I have to keep restraining myself with you. It's like I'm the father who wants to reach out a hand and help the child cross the stepping stones. I have to let the child slip and slide on his own though, because he has to experience the process himself.

"I know you are going a certain place and you have an inner knowledge of what your purpose is. But you get side-tracked and spin your wheels. You're looking for forms outside of yourself."

As we walked, we talked about how I could attract to myself the kind of work that I wanted--whatever that was. Gently, Jan Paul suggested that one place to start was with the way I dressed. He felt that I presented myself as too artsy and Bohemian, too unpowerful. He then offered himself and his friend, Marie, to "do a dressing." He'd studied "dressing" in San Francisco with Robert Pante, the author of *Dressing to Win*, and Marie knew fashion from her years at Nordstrom's Department store.

A few nights later Jan Paul and Marie arrived to start the "dressing" process. Jack happened to be in the kitchen repairing the sink, and he looked askance at me as he heard what they were going to do. They set to work like garbage wreckers pulling garments out of the closet and throwing them in huge plastic bags. For the most part it was easy to watch. The crowded, cluttered closet had oppressed me, but I'd lacked the personal wherewithal to clean it out and start from scratch.

Jan Paul pointed out, "These clothes keep you in the past." I agreed, especially since some of them had been with me since high school--20 years! (I just couldn't throw out that quality Pendleton skirt, even though I never wore it. ... I bought that dress in India. ...) But now I was evolving out of my business, out of my marriage, and out of the old behaviors. I had no wish to live in the past. At the same time, I had no wish to so completely re-fashion myself that I lost the freedom and comfort I enjoyed when wearing my fatigues or walking in my Birkenstocks.

It wasn't hard to let most of the clothes go. Having someone else do the drastic deed made it simple. The only stumbling block was my white cotton summer dress with the Chinese crocheted jacket. "It's too frilly," they said, "Too little girl. Too unpowerful."

Although I saw their point, I couldn't part with it just yet. It was one of the few outfits in which I'd received lavish compliments. When I wore it I felt wonderfully attractive and feminine and I didn't necessarily want to be powerful in it.

Jan Paul and Marie pretty well cleaned things out, leaving me with only a pair of slacks, one pair of jeans, two sweaters and two dresses. I felt unburdened, lighter. I relished looking at the empty space in the closet. Lifting one bag, I was amazed at the sheer weight of the clothes inside it. No wonder I felt lighter.

Jack beckoned me from the kitchen. He was concerned about the ruthlessness of the two image makers. He assured me, "You present yourself well, no matter what. Just take this all with a grain of salt." Thanking him for his concern and care, I assured him that I could handle it. I suspected he was also wondering how I planned to pay for the new influx of clothes. I wondered that myself.

Jan Paul said, "Look at that empty closet! The universe will rush in to fill the vacuum, you'll see. By going out on a limb, you're putting yourself in a place of receptivity. Instead of hanging on to old stuff until you create the new job and the money, you're creating the image now and through that, the job and the money will manifest themselves."

I believed him.

That night I slept poorly. Images of my depleted wardrobe floated in and out of my mind. In vain, I tried to picture myself wearing the remaining clothes day after day and making it all look good. Awakening early with still more clothes thoughts, I was tempted to retrieve a pair of grey shoes so that I'd at least have shoes for my two remaining dresses. But I resisted the urge. I truly was ready just to let the money and the clothes come as I generated the place and the prosperity for them.

> *"Change and growth take place when a person has risked himself and dares to become involved with experimenting with his own life." said Herbert Otto. To do this, to experiment with your own life, is very exhilarating, full of joy, full of happiness, full of wonder, and yet it's also spooky. It's also frightening because you are dealing with the unknown, and you are shaking complacency."*
>
> *Leo Buscaglia,* ***Living, Loving and Learning***

Several days later I again met with Jan Paul and Marie. For the first part of the evening the session was fairly standard. I tried on my surviving clothes and they suggested how to make them work. I had to eliminate my handwoven rose dress, acknowledging that it lacked fit and wasn't flattering, even though it was a work of art. They would have liked to eliminate the whole lot and start from scratch, but they knew I couldn't afford it.

Then we got to my hair. I'd been wearing it with a full bush of bangs and the rest pulled loosely back over my ears clasped behind my neck.

Jan Paul said, "It's too uneven, too shaggy."

Marie said, "I'd love to see you pull it back closer to the sides of your head."

"No way," I said, "I can't expose my ears because of my hearing aids."

This got us off on a whole new tangent--a process of learning all in itself. They questioned and prodded. Wouldn't I consider this new idea?

"Absolutely not. I simply won't wear a style that would show my hearing aids."

"Even if we, as your advisers, tell you that it would make you look a lot better?" they asked.

"Never. I think it looks cluttered. It obstructs the line of the ear to see that mechanical thing in there."

"What if you were paying us $1000 to advise you? Would you accept our advice?"

"Not even then," I insisted.

"Would you consider it if you knew it could make $600 a month difference in your pay check?" asked Jan Paul.

"No. I just don't think it looks good."

Then Marie offered, "You know, just now when I realized that you wear hearing aids, I stood back in surprise. I didn't know how I should respond. I guess because you never told me. Knowing it makes me feel closer to you. I feel aware of you in a more vulnerable way."

Jan Paul said, "You're covering up--hiding something. The whole point of the dressing is for people to get the real you, who you really are. It's actually dishonest for you not to just be. When you can wear your hair as you want and show the world who you are--with pride--than you will indeed make a powerful impact."

Marie asked, "What would be wrong with allowing people to know you as you are? It actually gives you *more* power. It gives you a place from which to make a more real impression. If people know you for who you are and know your hearing problem, they will have more compassion and respect for you--perhaps a stronger awareness of who you are."

So, in the process, I moved. I became excited about allowing myself to wear the flattering hair styles that this new concept introduced. I even got excited about the idea of just letting the world know. Let them recognize me for my honesty and for being real. After all, Katherine Hepburn was my model. *She* would do as she pleased and let the world take her as she was--and respect her all the more for it.

I had a very soft, outflowing feeling toward Jan Paul and Marie. They led me through the process so gently and without intimidating me. At the conclusion, I felt good and I really felt different. I'd discovered a new and different perspective. It felt right, and I liked it.

> *"Change is not easy, but it's absolutely unavoidable ... Growth accompanies positive changes; determining to risk the outcome resulting from a changed behavior or attitude will enhance our self-perceptions. We will have moved forward; in every instance our lives will be influenced by making a change that only each of us can make."*
>
> *from,* ***Each Day A New Beginning***

It seemed that one obstacle after another delayed the final step in the clothes process. Finally, after several weeks, the big day came. It was an important occassion because of the huge shift in my self-perception regarding clothes. I met Jan Paul and Marie at Mario's, a place so far removed from my standard shopping haunts that I didn't even know where it was. (It happened to be one of the trendiest boutiques in Portland.) I suppose it was appropriate that while I waited for three o'clock to arrive, I wandered into a resale store and browsed.

At Mario's, Jan Paul and Marie selected clothes entirely unlike what I would have chosen. Some major shifting of old patterns was required in order for me to be open to them. I strenuously objected to a cobalt-blue jersey skirt, telling them, "I never wear pleats from the waist. It emphasizes my stomach."

How surprised I was to see that I looked smashing in it. I still had a tummy, but it simply wasn't that noticeable, and certainly not worth denying myself that striking skirt.

Some of the clothes were fashionably awful, while certain ones looked really great. I had to admit that I looked terrific in them too. I just had to open myself to wearing them daily instead of on special occasions. I had to move myself away from the old concept of melting into the crowd to the new concept of standing out in the crowd--not garishly, but in a tasteful, elegant way.

Jan Paul and Marie only spent 45 minutes with me and then I stayed on to re-try everything one more time. After another hour and more re-trying, I finally plunked down $385 for one pair of cream silk pants, the cobalt skirt, a matching blue silk blouse and blue cardigan, and a turquoise pullover sweater.

Before pulling out my Visa card, I did a lot of figuring and organizing and planning. At last I let go of my fears. Money was going to have to flow out sooner or later, and I might as well get on with it. With that hurdle over, I then crossed the street to Nordstrom's and tried on more clothes. I was getting into the swing of this. I liked the new person I saw standing reflected in the mirror. I never dreamed I could look stylish and be comfortable at the same time.

At Nordstrom's I pushed myself even further out of my comfort zone. Agonizing over the considerations of practicality versus aesthetics, I chose the coat that looked the best--cream wool--instead of the one which was the most practical. It was a challenge and quite a stretch to imagine myself wearing a white coat and having it stay unsoiled and unsnagged.

I told myself, *I **can** open up to this working. I can wear this coat to work, City Club and concerts and it will be perfect.* Interesting--I already saw myself holding back from wearing it simply because I feared I'd look too overwhelming. I realized, *I have to open up to that being okay. It's not **bad** to look terrific.*

"As an individual transcends his limited self-idea, as he grows into a larger self by surrendering even some aspect of the fear which grips and cripples him, he gradually discovers that he can do what he previously believed he could not do ... this discovery--and the behaviors which ensue--amounts to an awakening."

Marsha Sinetar, ***Do What You Love, The Money Will Follow***

CHAPTER TWENTY

AT THE SAME time that the clothes process was underway, changes were also taking place in my work life. Only a few days after Jan Paul and Marie emptied my closets I had my first appointment with Victor Manning. He owned and ran the Whole Health Center, and I thought he might give me some guidance regarding my health problems. Victor was an incredibly energetic 62-year-old leprechaun--tall and wiry, white-haired with twinkling eyes, and moving all the time. The meeting with him set me on a new course.

When I arrived at the rambling old clinic, Victor beckoned me into the little cubicle of an exam room. He was seated on a stool at the foot of an exam table holding the feet of a woman lying on her back on the table. "I'm doing a reading on a woman in Connecticut," Victor said. "This is my helper, Joanne, and she's the surrogate body."

Victor would ask Joanne's body if such and such was good or bad for the patient. He would get a reading from the degree that her feet did or didn't line up.

It looked incredibly far-out, yet it was a procedure that was recommended and used by the author-doctor Lendon Smith and other physicians. Joanne, the lady on the table had, until recently, endured terrible candida symptoms very similar to mine. Now she was greatly improved.

When he finished with Joanne, Victor had me lie down on the table. There were many interruptions. People coming in and out.

Phone ringing. But gradually Victor attended to all the questions regarding my body. He showed me the first set of questions on a sheet of paper. A reading of zero indicated that the organ or gland or whatever in question was functioning at correct levels. The higher up the scale the number, the more out of whack the organ.

My hydrochloric acid was 10, meaning I lacked it to that degree. Acidophilus was 11. Adrenals were 9. Candida was 10. My aura was 4. It should have been in the 200 range. Victor said, "No wonder you feel tired. The amino acids are not getting through. Your body is just hanging in trying to keep going."

There were many other questions which he asked the body. Allergies were many. Nystatin, the medication which I'd taken in such quantities over the last year to kill the candida, was deadly for me, a 10.

Through the leg-length testing I asked Victor about other things. The answers: You should not do the Personal Effectiveness Seminar now. You will not get the benefit from it because your body is so run-down. You need to regenerate. PES is a very positive program. You should do it in June.

As soon as Victor recommended that I postpone PES I grew relieved. I'd had misgivings about such a strenuous five days. Now it looked as if I'd have the time beautifully set up for five days of healing instead. I'd already organized for the PES so I had no work at which I was expected, no guitar lessons for which to practice, no meetings. Now I was free to rest and rejuvenate, to be calm with whatever healing crises might be stirred up as I embarked on Victor's health program.

My concern was how I would explain it to Jan Paul. I feared that he would go into a pissy funk about how I was delaying my enlightenment. I didn't look forward to his cross examining or his "I love you and it makes me sad when you spin your wheels and stay stuck."

Lately it seemed that Jan Paul was playing the devil's advocate, and not in the gentle supportive manner he originally had. Now I detected his impatience. He was less willing to lead or guide me through processes. *Perhaps he is just sick of processes anyway,* I told myself, *since he's doing them all the time in his work.*

In response to issues I brought up he would say, "Wait till you've done the PES," or "I see you as the person you will become," or "I see you when you're in touch with your power," and then, "You're still stuck in your stuff. I'm impatient that you're not moving ahead faster."

So was I.

But I had to pay attention to me. Although I wanted to do the PES and I wanted Jan Paul's approval, I needed to first get on with the business of healing. I knew I had to be more strict with my diet. I knew my body was run-down and tired. The puffiness, the bloating, the inability to sleep, the nervousness, the cravings, the insatiable appetite, the flabbiness and fogginess, the hip pain, all these problems had to be handled. It was easy for Jan Paul to stand on the sidelines and criticize my explorations and programs in healing. He didn't live with a body that was unresponsive, that wouldn't function as it should. He slept easily, had no cravings. He worked out.

A week later I had my second exam session with Victor. One of my questions, via the leg length testing, was, "Does Victor need someone to work for him?" I propositioned, "Wouldn't you like to go home before eight o'clock in the evening?" He obviously needed someone to answer the phone, receive patients, and unpack and organize the supplements.

"I know I can help you," I told him. "I have an excellent business, organizational background and, goodness knows, I'm an expert on candida."

Victor said, "You're too high-powered." (Meaning, I was sure, that he'd have to pay me too much.)

I responded, "I'll work in exchange for treatment in the beginning. As I become more of an asset for you, you can pay me money."

So it was decided. I wondered, *Is this the step, the link, I've been moving toward?* It was so perfect for me. I had experienced all the candida symptoms first-hand. I'd read and gathered endless information on it. My own experience and my nutritional reading meant that I could offer so much. I realized, *I **can** positively affect the women who come in, I **can** make a difference ... working holistically with women just as the psychic last month predicted.*

I could actually see my dream coming true--of being a helpmate to a practitioner who already had the structure. The Whole Health Center bulged with piles of nutrition books, newsletters, all kinds of information. Doctors were constantly phoning and dropping in and out. The client ahead of me that day had been utterly boggled by the onslaught of candida information Victor showered on her. I told her to phone me if she needed guidance or support, and Victor encouraged her to do so. It all seemed so natural.

Two weeks later at Jan Paul's, I noticed that he'd removed the photo of me and Woo, which he'd kept on his desk for three months. Sadly, I admitted to myself that the closeness and the delight were pretty much gone. Why? Did I get so wrapped up in my own life? Did he in his? Simply lack of time? I was less needy of him and he of me. I was critical of him and he of me. I had feelings come up of irritation, obligation and annoyance toward him. I was sure the same came up for him.

I missed the interaction. When we did get together, I was annoyed at Jan Paul's quizzings: "What's up? What did you do today?" Lately it seemed that he heard me say whatever I did and he was partly, silently judging and partly, not even listening. No more deep, smiling gazes at me. No more reinforcements of my power and beauty. No more phone calls. No more visits or wanting to get together in an evening. The change had accelerated after I saw Victor. When I'd cancelled the PES. Jan Paul perceived me as "doing what you want anyway," and as having some deep dark subconscious motive in postponing the PES. He just had to take it personally and to make his private judgments of me.

"Whatever you do, SOMEONE won't approve. SOMEONE will resist your changes. Don't let that stop you. Your life is YOURS."
Read and Rusk, ***I Want to Change, But I Don't Know How***

My days at the Whole Health Clinic were exciting and full. I felt truly in my element. Numerous people called with complaints or questions. When Victor wasn't there to handle it, they accepted my counsel. The first time a patient phoned feeling sluggish and depressed, I flashed, "Oh boy! This is my chance!" Momentarily I hesitated, wondering, *Am I ready for this? Do I have the ability to help her along?* But it was only for a moment. Then I plunged into the process and never looked back.

With her, and with others, I spent a long time on the phone giving lots of guidance and information on detoxifying and what not to eat. After I'd helped one lady via the phone, she later that day came into the clinic and we talked some more. Propitiously, Victor rang from

London while she was there. How wonderfully validating it was to have him give her the same information I had.

All day long people phoned who needed help with their allergy or candida programs. Patients came in overwhelmed with the challenge of preparing meals for themselves or for their spouses, some of whom either had different allergies than theirs or none at all. I would offer ideas and let them express their frustrations.

As these people came and went I felt fully in my power. So centered, so at my source, so *effective*. I could see the process developing me and leading me to classes and counseling and teaching. *Each patient helps me solidify my foundation,* I told myself. *My ability grows and so does my awareness of the questions and the needs of each one.*

"We teach what we want to learn."
Anonymous

After one particularly chock-a-block day, I drove home glowing. I was keenly aware that it was interaction with people that made my life meaningful. After each experience of the day I'd thought, "That was great!" I loved the counseling, informing, the consciousness-raising of those who came in or phoned the clinic. It was so easy, because I'd been in the same place of fear and weakness, just as they now were.

The day had been typically action-packed. I had organized Victor's pill room, typed answers to inquiries, attended City Club for Victor (looking wonderful in my new clothes) and helped puzzled patients with questions about the program. Before coming home I went to the weekly macrobiotic dinner and then attended my singing teacher's concert. Only after I got home, did I pause to appreciate the day's activities. It seemed incredible to realize that I actually did it all--and it never occurred to me to question my endurance.

From the dark of my bedroom I gazed out at the satin sheen of the moon illuminating the roofs and trees. I lifted my voice in thanksgiving for the joyful day, for my living it fully, for the delight of the people and the moments. There was nothing I lacked. I was happy and complete. I thought, ***I** am a miracle!* More and more I came into touch with that awareness. Standing by the window in the moonlight, I was filled with the wonder of such completeness and well-being. *There is a power there--within me--and I take my baby steps to accepting it and not fearing or backing away from it.*

> *"True self love is ... an intimate act between you and yourself. Self love seems to unlock this storehouse of divine love. You find compassion for your human weaknesses and the tenderness spreads to others."*
>
> *Read and Rusk,* ***I Want to Change, But I Don't Know How***

My work at the Center so stimulated me that I decided to go back to school in order to earn a master's degree in counseling. Typically, I was impatient to get on with it, and, although my days were already full to bursting, I enrolled in an evening class at Marylhurst College.

The first evening I drove straight from work to my relationship class. Once settled into the lecture hall, for the first time I recognized the enormity of what I was undertaking. With surprise, I began to comprehend that I had to write papers, define goals, analyze, quote references, read sources. All of which I wanted to do. Yet I saw that the time commitment would mean that other areas in my life would have to be cut back. I wasn't accustomed to classroom deadlines, disciplines ... although what had I done all those years in business, but handle deadlines and be disciplined? Suddenly the idea of a grade sent internal anxieties careening through my body. I had to perform!

But at least I would perform with style! Earlier that afternoon I had represented the Whole Health Center at the Chamber of Commerce, and I had met people whom I'd not seen for over a year. I had worn my new blue outfit and had actually felt very comfortable doing so. People had said, "You look great," and "Whatever you are doing agrees with you." I *felt* powerful and effective and expressed myself accordingly.

By the time I arrived at Marylhurst for my class, I was far beyond being self-conscious about my clothes. Instead, I felt totally appropriately dressed--*well* dressed, and not out of place. I was growing more and more uncomfortable in the old clothes--more and more aware of how they didn't work for me. Just like the past.

The clothes process had been an outer reflection of the inner beliefs which once limited me. The habits of negativity and of seeking approval, of expecting rejection if I looked too good, of avoiding risk-taking or standing out in a crowd, the concern that I would ruin nice clothes on the first outing, and the apprehension about revealing my hearing loss to the world--i.e. the fear of being vulnerable--were all patterns with which Jan Paul and the clothes process had confronted me. The experience had forced me to grow and change. In order to wear the new clothes, I'd literally suspended old patterns. The beauty of changing myself through changing my clothes was that I received immediate feedback on whether or not the change was working, on whether or not I liked the change. Without exception, the verbal feedback, the new ways I felt and acted, as well as the image in the mirror, brilliantly reflected the desirability of accepting and embracing those changes.

> *"In the process of defining myself, I have a tendency to set up rules and boundaries and then forget that rules are made to be broken, as are boundaries to be expanded and crossed."*
>
> *Joanna Field, from* ***Each Day a New Beginning***

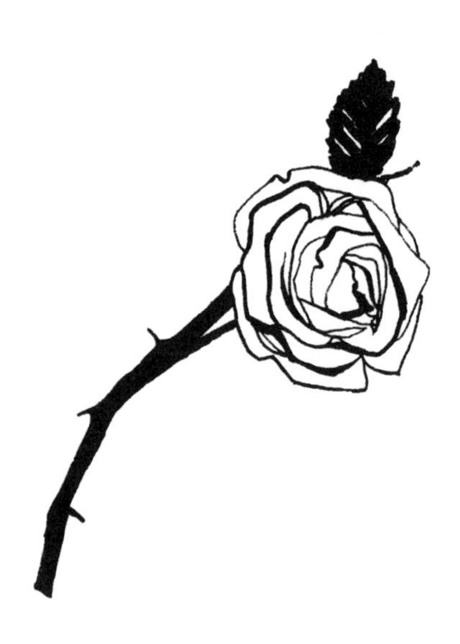

CHAPTER TWENTY ONE

MY ABILITY TO exercise was such an up and down condition. One day I regaled friends with the triumphs of my new energy and my strong body. Then the next day I found my energy level slipping and sinking down and down until I was so low that I could barely struggle home after work and collapse into bed.

There were days like the sunny Saturday when I raked leaves. Each time I climbed the stairs or pushed the wheelbarrow uphill I wondered if I'd feel "normal" at the top. Arriving there, experiencing no residue of the climb, no weakness, no achiness--I'd be surprised--surprised that my legs didn't give out, ache, or go numb. I'd lost touch with what it was like to experience normal bodily activities.

At some point I had stopped fearing overdoing as Dr. Swank had warned me. I now viewed each and every movement, every physical activity as *only* beneficial, as a necessary part of the healing process. I had gradually arrived at the conclusion that I, alone, must determine the course of my healing. I could look to doctors for information and guidance, but, ultimately, only I could decide what approach was right for me. Releasing my yearning to rely on others, particularly experts, was an important step, but oh, so difficult.

I continued gleaning everything I could from reading. One book inspired me to try a new form of visualization--speaking aloud what I wanted to visualize. I took my cue from Catherine Ponder's statement in *The Dynamic Laws of Healing*, that the spoken word is 80% more effective than the thought word or written word. At first it was difficult to come up with the phrases I wanted and to say them smoothly. Once I started, however, the words flowed almost of their own accord. I verbally praised my sturdy, healthy legs and gave thanks for my strong muscles, constitution and my healed body, for every cell that was filled with the positivism that infused my body ... etc.

I was surprised at the power of the chant-like flow of words. It was an exercise in having to formulate the thoughts into verbal entities and that *forced me to think clearly* and to focus on what I wanted. The verbal expression of thought definitely deepened my awareness of what I wanted. It was as if the words infused a power of their own, as if the act of constructing them had built a new structure.

In mid-March I was feeling strong enough to participate in a Vision Expansion seminar that Jan Paul presented. Little did I dream how far reaching those three days would be. The seminar was powerful and wonderful. Each day burst with movement into new frameworks and was full of interacting, loving and becoming acquainted with special people. I learned about myself and dropped some old beliefs, and emerged from the weekend feeling exhilarated.

I was renewed in my love and admiration for Jan Paul--for his skill, talent and heart shining through, and for his intellect and articulation. I wondered how I had allowed myself to slip so far out of touch with such a man. It seemed hard to believe that we had ever spent such an intimate six months together.

I noticed the parts of the seminar which had evolved from some of our times together ... the Rampal music that I gave him ... the Slight Edge illustrations ... the learning about being unattached. I took a certain pleasure in knowing I'd played a role in his evolution to this point.

All the while I watched Victor, whom I'd coerced into coming, and I beamed each time I saw him mellowing and opening up, sharing and enjoying. And on Sunday, there was Karl, whose first word to me was "Definitely." We were sitting on the floor, knee to knee, and Jan Paul was guiding us to look deeply into our partner's eyes and notice the beauty there. I saw something--a depth, a charge, a command, a softness. There was something powerful that happened in that exchange. I felt drawn inexorably to Karl, focusing only on one thing--that I wanted very much to be held long and close by this man and to hold and hug him over and over.

Throughout the remainder of the day I was keenly aware of this tall, handsome man. I listened especially attentively to his sharings, and I was drawn even more to him because of the sensitive, poetic way he expressed himself. How insightful and perceptive he was of the people and of the experience we were all in. Increasingly, I knew I wanted to be with him, to know him. I managed to go for lunch with him and two women--all four of us wearing our double eye patches and looking like people in x-rated pictures who have their eyes blocked out. We received many quizzical glances from other diners.

When the seminar was over, I lingered on, waiting for the chance when we could be together without everyone intercepting us. Karl had women buzzing around him like bees to a honey jar. I had no hesitation or shyness, and simply asked him, "Could we talk before you leave?" I *knew* he wanted to connect with me too.

We went to dinner at Rax's and got acquainted over a salad bar meal, then went home together to watch "Jewel in the Crown" while he massaged my back. We cuddled and talked and became quite passionate, and I was amazed that something I'd dreamed had so easily manifested itself. It came from the purposeful expectation. It couldn't help but happen, I'd been so clear about my desire and my undoubting expectations that it would indeed take place. I guess I was a little surprised that the reality of my vision had come about so quickly.

We made love till two in the morning. I delighted in being with such a virile, big, strong man, one who was decisive and powerful, yet tender and expressive. I was amazed at myself, too, realizing that I was enjoying being with a man who was only 29 years old. In some ways I noticed the age difference, but in the enjoyment of each other it made no difference. I felt we both had learning to do from each other.

"In praise of older women ... " he said.

A week later I had my first date with Karl. We talked non-stop throughout the evening, at dinner, and later walking in the park. I'd think, "Wow. This is interesting," or "Isn't it incredible that we are not at a loss for words."

More dates followed, but not too often. Every week or so Karl would drive up from his home in Salem. I loved walking arm in arm with him. He was the tallest man I'd ever been with (such a contrast with Jan Paul who was the shortest!) and it was a wonderful feeling to be so dwarfed, to have the sense of myself being petite and feminine next to him. He liked my body--thought it was amazing for my age, and said, "You look half as old from your neck down. It's only from your neck up that you look 40."

Another time he observed, "You're one of those women who is always attractive, who men put on a pedestal."

In the old days I had certainly never perceived myself as attractive. I saw myself so now, though, and that was what he took his perception from.

He said, "I fantasize taking Jack aside and telling him how he should have been with you so that you both could have had good sex."

How sweet that the younger man could feel that he had advice for Jack. The beauty was that he did ... Karl was so open to learning what was necessary and so keenly aware of my needs as a woman. He'd understood perfectly when I explained about the herpes, reassuring me that a little problem like the herpes virus needn't disrupt our intimacy. He said that he completely trusted me to tell him should we be together when I had an outbreak--which fortunately seemed to be rare.

I loved his picking me up and carrying me into the bedroom, loved the way he sometimes treated me like a young girl ... as when he insisted that I practice getting in and out of his sports car with the high tech seat belt on.

He said, "Sometimes I feel older than you are."

Maybe it was not age so much as it was his feeling more competent in certain areas. His attitude came across sweet and protective. I felt looked after, feminine, girlish. Ahhh! I suddenly realized that what I was learning from Karl was how to play ... how to let the child in me be in a relationship. I thought of activities that would be fun to share with him ... I wanted to slide down the hydrotube at Washington Square. I wanted to go dancing, to movies, to play racquetball! *And I will!* I told myself. *I want to hike, to raft ... to have fun!*

I didn't want to live with Karl or to have a serious deep involvement. We could talk about deeper things and concepts. *But*, I realized, *the **fun** is the lesson.*

One time Karl said, "You're like a 16-year-old girl. You blush. You get embarrassed when I look at you."

That child-like, girlish part of me had not surfaced at all with Jack or Peter or in all my day-to-day interactions. I had touched on it a little bit with Jan Paul. That girlish part--the person who was light hearted and enjoyed being picked up or held down or tickled, who liked to do things not for their social or business value, the girl who liked to blush and feel that she was not the controller in the relationship--that was the part of me that I was renewing my acquaintance with. I had hardly known it existed. Certainly it had been squirreled away for years.

> *"The child is an almost universal symbol for the soul's transformation. The child is whole, not yet divided ... When we would heal the mind ... we ask this child to speak to us."*
>
> *Susan Griffin, from* ***Each Day a New Beginning***

Whenever Karl rang, I was pleased to hear from him and then would be astounded when, an hour later, we would hang up. It seemed surprising that we could have so much to talk about. Among other things, we talked about sex and orgasms, about his mother and religion, and about his goals and concerns in relationships. His insight was very attuned, very sensitive--especially for a young man. I had no inhibitions about talking to him, and I believed I learned from him by the questions he raised.

The sex was delightful, but I especially loved the talking and the sharing. Most of the time it was two-way. We explored ideas and thoughts together ... particularly issues which Karl brought up. But they were thoughts that I was interested in learning more about too. What *did* I expect from relationships? What did I want out of ours? Did I want to invest in a relationship that wasn't long term?

I had no doubt that my relationship with Karl was not long term. Even so, I noticed the fears cropping up when I thought of him no longer driving up from Salem to see me ... when I thought of him pulling back so he could spend more time with the attractive girls he was bound to meet. I was aware that I definitely wanted a quality sexual relationship in my life. *Perhaps just knowing it will keep them coming*, I reassured myself. *When Karl is gone there will be others.*

Sometimes my thoughts would flit ahead to when I would meet my predicted soulmate. It seemed inconceivable that there was a soulmate or partner for me. I felt so very complete as I was. I basked in the glow and warmth of the widening circle of friends in my life. My times with Karl happened only every other week or so. When he wasn't there, I was content and happy after work, to retire home to my quiet sanctuary and to share my alone times with the cats.

I had no sense of lack because there was no all-encompassing partner. It seemed incredible for me to consider that a man could exist about whom I could feel that way. I was so pleased with the men who were already around me. In fact I was a bit surprised to notice that I was continually in contact with sensitive, powerful, gentle men ... Jan Paul, Karl, Peter, Victor, the men from the workshops and the macrobiotic dinners. ... Certainly most, except for Karl, were just "hello" acquaintances. But I felt the good feelings they had about me, and I had no desire or need for more than that.

One night I dreamed I was lying in the arms of my soulmate and was completely encircled in love and protection. When I awoke I missed him and wanted to be with him again. How strange and how different this was for me. I'd not had a sense of *wanting* him--anyone--at all, until that moment.

I meditated, giving thanks for this unknown mate. The sense of his presence was deeply etched in my memory. Suddenly I was overwhelmingly, piercingly filled with the perception of my own power. It was as if my soulmate gave me that message in my dream. Tears streamed down my face as I gave thanks for the process that had led me to the awareness of myself and of this inner power. And then I was struck by the level of acceptance I'd achieved. I whispered to myself, *I know there is something in me that is powerful. I say yes! to allowing that power to shine forth.*

The moment was profound. *I **know** I am a healer, a teacher, an inspiration, one who raises the consciousness of those I contact. I **know** I have the power to heal and uplift and to teach and to love.* I felt awed. I said out loud, *I **accept** the power. No more apologizing. No more fears. No more suppression. No more anxiety.* I felt filled through and through with the consciousness of that power *and* the acceptance of it. Step by step I had moved toward this recognition, experiencing bits and pieces of it over the preceding months. Somehow that morning it was as if I'd been struck by lightning. I realized, *I am there. I am* ***in*** *it. I* ***am*** *it.*

There was no looking back. Only the joy of the discovering; the thrill of the awareness that indeed I ***was*** a powerful woman, and indeed I had arrived at an acceptance of my power.

I asked myself, *Did all this come from the dream?*

Moments of such awareness would occur. And then I would forget. As I expressed it in those times, I didn't know what was really meant. Now I perceive that the qualities that I began to get in touch with were not exclusive to me, but are universal to all of us, and they shine forth in the degree we are open to them. I was becoming aware not of "my" power, but of "the" power/source/Self --whatever one wants to call it. But how quickly those recognitions would slip away.

> *"You know quite well, deep within you, that there is only a single magic, a single power, a single salvation ... and that is called loving."*
>
> *Herman Hesse*

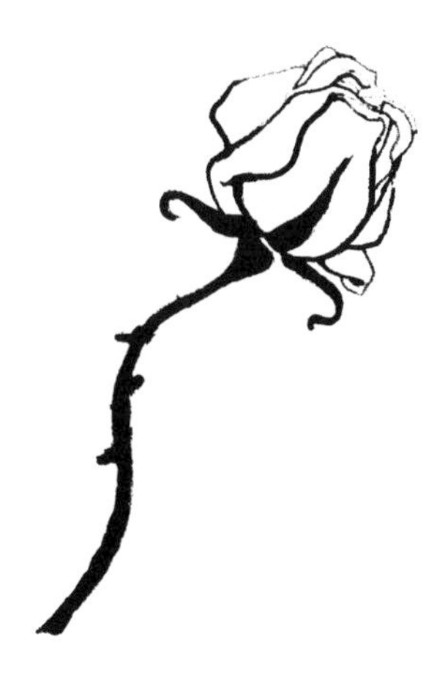

CHAPTER TWENTY TWO

AT THE WEEKLY macrobiotic dinners which I attended, I met a man who would play a pivotal role in my transformation process. Steve Hillinger, a tall, robust man with a gentle, yet penetrating manner, was a counselor and a teacher in many ways. One way was as a leader of firewalks. When he first told me about the firewalks I was deeply drawn to experiencing them under his guidance. A part of me knew that I had the capability. Yet another part of me undercut it with my fears. My body grew tight and tense whenever I thought about actually firewalking. As Steve pointed out, though, "The body is in a state of excitement, and you can view that positively or negatively."

I believed that once having done firewalking I could then do anything. I saw it as a valuable tool for learning to access my inner power. I felt that I didn't tap that power often--that I actually feared tapping it. I was afraid of what I would--or wouldn't--let loose, of what works I might set in motion or that I'd fail to meet the challenge. *Of course the results will be positive,* I told myself. Yet I was afraid.

I also believed that firewalking would yield control. That I would be able to remember walking the fire and I'd be able to calm down, or meditate, or sleep, at will. It would be a lesson in trust--an experience of total Self/God trust. The image I'd always held was that one had to be a holy man in India to accomplish firewalking. Yet I knew that I had the same capability as that holy man. I too was a "holy man." Steve's wife, Brenda, who was a producer for Channel

8, and who was sophisticatedly attractive with make-up and red fingernails, had firewalked nine times. Admiring her from across the table at the macrobiotic dinners, I imagined what fears she must have overcome and what self-trust she must experience in her life.

Images of the firewalk simmered in my mind, and I wished that I could discuss my fears and feelings with someone. Then one Saturday my need was met. I awoke with a sticky sore throat. Even so, I saw no reason not to forge ahead with all the doingness activities I had scheduled for the day. I had contracted to do a huge wedding order, so I hurried across town to the flower market. As soon as I arrived there, though, my energy went zap-o and I felt terrible. My head said, *Accomplish your wedding order ... Fulfill your agreement with Carol this afternoon and go practice a duet.* My body said, *Rest.* My ego said, *I want to share my singing at the party Sunday*. I weighed the choices and finally decided, *Listen to my body*, and drove home and sank into bed.

As I rested the phone rang. It was Amata, the beautiful Hawaiian woman I'd met at Jan Paul's vision seminar. How wonderful it was to talk to her. I perceived her presence as that of a true Woman Warrior--as an earth goddess who brought contact with the deep heart of women and whose wisdom would be a catalyst for me.

I talked to her about firewalking. Interestingly, her family history was of living at the base of Mt. Pele. Every time it erupted her family's lands were spared. Her family name meant "daughter of the fire."

She explained to me, "The fire is purification. You carry the gold within you. It is surrounded by the black dross. When you walk through fire it is not the gold that is burned, but the dross--you fear getting burned, but more importantly you fear that you will discover there is no gold."

How true. How wisely put. My fear revolved around arriving at the walk site and undermining my power to walk through the fire. Yet I knew without doubt, deep within me, that I indeed had the capability to firewalk. Had I not already demonstrated that I had the capacity to heal, to draw the man I wanted to me, to make a candle flame flicker or burn steadily? Yet I still doubted. Because frequently, when I was not deeply in touch with my believing, in my trusting, then I couldn't control the candle flame, or so many other things within myself.

Because I continued to undermine my power, that was exactly the reason for walking. I longed to embrace and employ that power source immediately. Why should I take twenty years to access it when I could confront my fears head-on, and thus move forward in my life with that power known and available to me right away?

I thought about how wonderful it would be to tell Mom and Dad and others that I had firewalked. And I knew that was a very wrong reason for walking. It was ego again. And I feared that the ego would get in the way when the time came. That I'd be poised to walk and the ego would want so much to experience walking that it would fear that, therefore, it wouldn't, and then indeed I wouldn't.

Amata said, "You've already experienced hell, your individual walk through the fire. Now it is time for you to manifest it literally."

Amata's phone call was singularly timely. As I put down the phone, I thought how there were no coincidences in life. No accidents or flukes.

"Fire is the test of gold ..."
Seneca, ***Moral Essays***

I hadn't heard from Jan Paul in several weeks. Then one day he phoned, glowing and bubbling. "I'm in love!" he gushed. "With Kathy from the Vision seminar ... I feel like a teenager ... She's a Scorpio ... She's so fragile ... Her life works ... she's powerful ... I want to protect her and support her and would do anything for her ... I'm your friend. I don't know if we can still be lovers ..."

Even though I was unattached, something dropped within me as I sensed my loss. I recognized that the purpose of Jan Paul and me as lovers had perhaps been served. The time had come to open the space for whatever/whoever was necessary and important at this new stage.

Interestingly, my first thought was of phoning Karl ... or any other man. As if I craved male closeness and consolation now that Jan Paul was withdrawing that part of our relationship. How thankful I was to have gentle Betty tenderly looking into my eyes--and then she returned to her fastidious grooming.

To take my thoughts off Jan Paul, I gave myself the gift of a restful day--sunning on the patio and doing school work, appreciating the abundant verdure of the garden. The tulips, daffodils and hyacinths were blooming full blast. Their fragrance and that of the clematis assailed me each time I passed through the yard. I read the incoherent jumble of unrelated double talk which was part of my relationship class and I wondered, *Why I am doing this?*

Although I loved my work at the Whole Health Clinic and all my other activities, the pace of my life had been recklessly accelerating. As I allowed myself to get caught up in the whirl of trying to do too many things, events were beginning to control me rather than vice versa. My days congealed in a state of disarray. I hurried off in the morning and straggled in at night. At home I squeezed out enough energy to do one more thing and then collapsed into bed. There was never time to relax or catch up and the pile of undone demands climbed higher every day.

I knew exactly what was happening. I was being carried along on the same kind of drive and vigor and efficiency that had characterized the old Barbara. This scared me. There was an important lesson here: *It is to be calm, to be quiet, right in the middle of the busyness. It is essential that I learn how to tap only my energy and talent and to leave the pushing, racing, compulsive Barbara behind.*

I asked myself, *Is it possible for me to learn how to be slow-paced, calm, at peace, and in touch with my inner source* ***without*** *requiring constant reminders from my body?* More than ever, I appreciated the gift which my crashed body had given me. It had compelled me to recognize the desirability of dropping old habits and expectations, of letting go of trying to control the outer picture, and of learning, instead, to rely on my inner self.

There was another feature of the busyness that further drained me --that of pushing myself to do things I didn't enjoy. Instead of resting at night, I worked on flower orders in the frigid garage. Instead of attending to my school assignments, I made ribbon roses and garlands whenever I sat down for a "quiet" moment. Instead of taking time for myself, I filled each minute of the day with chores. None of my private life was being attended to, either businesswise or pleasurewise. Even though I hated doing the flower orders, I still hung on to Bloomers--for the money. It was obvious that I had to let it go, that I had to move on to the new, that I had to trust.

An incident occurred one evening which brought the confused whirl of my life into focus. It was like receiving a tap on the shoulder from the universe, a hand-delivered message. That night as I raced away from Marylhurst College after my classes, thinking only of getting home so I could eat, I was stopped by a policeman and given a speeding ticket.

My driving was like a metaphor for my life--speeding skillfully, but unaware. I was completely surprised when the policeman showed up behind me. I had no idea that I'd been speeding. I immediately realized that this was a pertinent message, "SLOW DOWN, BE AWARE." Who knows? That incident could perhaps have saved my life.

I couldn't help thinking how nice it would have been if I had an understanding partner to lovingly remind me to slow down, to take care of myself. But I realized, *That thought is coming from a place of weakness. The point is for* ***me*** *to learn to do that without assistance.* I had to access that awareness and ability within myself. The universe reminded me via my body. I had to learn to be attentive inwardly and not rely on the body or someone else to force me to it. As someone said:

"It only takes one person to change your life--you."
from, ***Each Day a New Beginning***

Later that night I lay on the bed listening to my Eileen Caddy tape. I'd heard it hundreds of times, but now I focused on her question, "Are you willing to move into the new? To cast off from the old life lines?"

Yes! Yes!--Then why don't I just do it?

Leaping out of bed, I hurried to the phone. I called Carol and canceled our singing practice. I rang Sara and roused her out of bed. She was even-voiced and non-blaming. She just said, "Shall we stop doing the Bloomers?"

"Yes! Yes!"

"Sleep on it," she said. A sharp lady. I had flipped back and forth so much during the last year. I knew why too. I had been going against the truth. My inner knowing had been telling me to stop the flower business. My money-worried outer voice kept exhorting me to hang on. My Hazelden book helped me remember:

"A new door cannot open until we've closed one behind us. The important fact is that a new one will always open without fail ... The pain of the old experience is trying to push us to new challenges, new opportunities, new growth."

Four days later I handled that "old" part of my life that was not working. It just came out--without more stewing and flip-flopping. I told Sara that I was truly ready to quit Bloomers. So was she. We both felt good about it.

"Each change is a 'little death'--an end to the old and a birth of the new. What does survive is our spirit, our willingness to grow."
Read and Rusk, ***I Want to Change, But I Don't Know How***

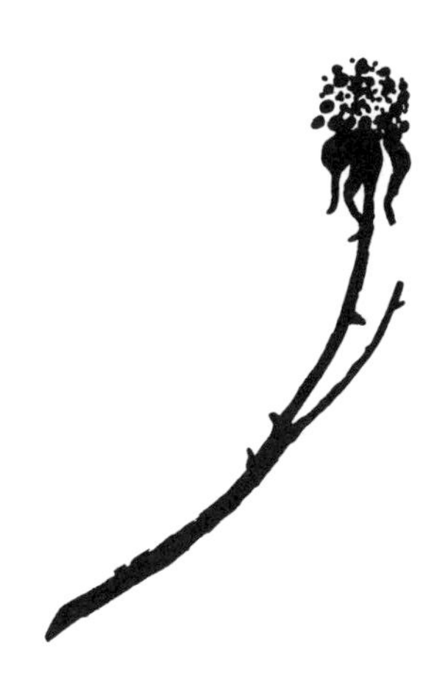

CHAPTER TWENTY THREE

ONE SUNNY AFTERNOON in late April I received a surprise phone call at the Whole Health Clinic. My sister in Santa Cruz, had grim news for me. Besides the leukemia, my father also had "blood on the brain" and needed to have brain surgery. Sis said, "The doctor gives him 50-50."

The next morning on the south-bound plane, I thought about my father, *a man who was and is and one day will not be.* I'd always known I would make this trip, and there was no heavy-handed emotion. I'd been confronted with Dad's mortality ever since he contracted the leukemia. On my lap lay the box of supplements Victor had sent with me. I felt so helpless to influence Dad to take them. Perhaps the point of the pills was not so much that I believed he would take them and they would help him, as much as it was my own need to feel I was doing something--anything. What else could I do? I could at least bring an offering of pills.

When I arrived in Santa Cruz, my sister told me that when Dad had awakened that morning and the nurse told him that he'd had brain surgery, he responded, "It's about time."

It was late afternoon when Mom, Sis and I entered the Intensive Care Unit at the hospital. Dad was sitting up. A white stocking cap covered his shaved head. His face was wan. He could talk, though it was hard to understand him without his teeth. With a hint of a twinkle in his eyes, he croaked, "Bring over some Cold Duck so I can wash down this medication."

I settled into the guest room in the hillside Santa Cruz house. It was such a pleasure to gaze down the smooth green slopes of the rolling pasture to the unblemished beauty of the coastal area. My heart went out to my father for having initiated the sale of his little empire right at that time. I imagined how he must have looked out of his window upon that land and been so content. Surely he would have preferred having no buildings constructed there while he still lived in his house.

Yet he had initiated the property sale and had maintained a supervisory role throughout. Was it hard, I wondered, to do it, knowing how his actions would lead to change that he couldn't possibly enjoy? He'd known, I was sure, that his life was beginning to set definable limits. Inwardly I thanked him for taking charge of the sale. None of the rest of the family had the taste nor the head for it. How wonderful it had been to have Dad to look after us once again--in yet another matter.

I believed that Dad's business affairs and his need to take care of the family were positive influences. They were the enticements that pulled him along. I speculated that he might be lying half awake in his hospital bed, dimly deciding whether or not to gather the resources to keep on, or to just slip gracefully away. On my final night in Santa Cruz I had the feeling that Dad had finally made his decision. His sense of responsibility to Mom and Sis, and to my brother and me was too strong. He wouldn't leave us as long as he felt he was capable of taking care of us.

Before I departed for the airport I saw Dad alone. It was a good leave-taking. I gently introduced the idea that he could heal himself and that I'd return soon. I talked about being positive and visualizing the blood and brain cells getting stronger, healthier and redder.

I said, "I'm sending you lots of positive vibrations."

He said, "You better keep them for yourself."

"I have enough for both of us ... I'm a strong lady. I--we--all love you and are so pleased you are getting better." Why was it so hard for me to say?

I could have cried then, and I could have cried again on the airplane. I was filled with the melancholy at our impending loss. *Who will take care of me?* I wondered. *Who will ever love me enough to look after me to the degree that Dad has done? I've taken it so for granted.*

"Don't be dismayed at good-byes. A farewell is necessary before you can meet again. And meeting again, after moments or lifetimes, is certain for those who are friends."

Richard Bach, ***Illusions***

Back in Portland, I had to address my frantic pace of life. There were so many activities that I wanted to do, but my body was dragging, demanding me to slow down. Obviously, I had to make some changes, but how I resisted doing so. I phoned Jan Paul and asked him to come over so I could use him as a sounding board.

"I hate my body this way," I said to Jan Paul.

"What would happen if you loved it this way?"

He helped me see that I *could* love it "this way." That I would sincerely enjoy the resting and the slower pace of life toward which my body was directing me.

He asked, "How many times do you have to be hit by a 2 x 4 in order to accept what you're being told? Clearly this isn't the path for you. You're being told you're not on the right track yet."

Tears were streaming down my face and I was hugging Gherkin to my chest. I wanted so much to do school *and* the Whole Health Center. It was clear that I had to make another choice--one or the other. The body wouldn't let me do both.

"I hate to let go of the Federal Loan."

"You'll get another."

"I hate to drop out of the program."

"You can hand papers in later."

"I want to be taken care of--"

"Back to that! You won't ask you're ex-husband to take care of you?"

We dropped that subject.

He said, "So you don't cure MS ... So you don't cure the candida ... You can either be happy or unhappy, fight it or not fight it."

"To be upset over what you don't have is to waste what you do have."

Ken Keyes Jr., ***The Handbook to Higher Consciousness***

The next morning, I awakened early, annoyingly sleepy, stiff and achy. But I awoke realizing that Jan Paul was right--evidently the route I'd picked wasn't the one the universe wanted for me. I was off track. But what was the *right* track? The one clear message was: Cut back.

I meditated, and from that the idea grew to let Victor decide. Either I'd work fewer days a week at the Whole Health Center and continue with school, or I'd work full time for Victor and quit school. Then I began to notice how good it felt to think the unthinkable; to acknowledge that it was okay for me to be late and incomplete with my exams and papers. Nothing drastic would happen. I could still get credit. I just wouldn't do it right away. It was okay! I noticed how good it felt to know I could come home and pursue the nutrition, meditation and other subjects that I'd been postponing so that I could handle school work.

I thought, *Whew! This is wonderful. Now that I've allowed myself to let go of the school I feel incredibly lighter.* I had wanted the school, and, for whatever reasons, that was not the correct route. School had meant a full-time two to three year commitment, which I could now see was too overburdening for me. Too restrictive. Too much limitation. Having accepted the idea of letting go, I felt fabulously free. At last I could concentrate on the workshops and the firewaking, the Hakomi body-mind therapy, the Neurolinguistic Programing, iridology ... reading ... cooking ... friends ... quiet times.

I must be letting go of the left brain concept of learning, I thought to myself. I recognized the value of reading for school and writing the papers. In earlier years, I'd enjoyed school work so much that the honors and degrees had practically been by-products. But the truth was that I was now happier learning experientially through the seminars and through my relating with people. I realized that I could completely release the traditional method of schooling. I could take courses and learn from them. But it wasn't necessary to do the papers or the projects or exams--because I couldn't help but learn anyway. The hours of homework (just like the flower shop) had taken me much too much away from my real goal--which was to be whole within myself and to interact with people out of that place of wholeness.

Certainly it was anguishing to give up the loan money that I so laboriously pursued and had finally received from the college. When I thought of the countless difficulties and the hours of filling out financial aid forms, I hated to turn it down. But, as Jan Paul said,

"You can always get another."

How much more balanced I felt once I made the decision to simply flow with what I could do at school, to not worry about fulfilling the deadlines and the requirements. I reassured myself that this was not simple copping out, laziness, lack of substance. My whole being felt so buoyant--I knew it was right.

> *"I always tell my students, go where your body and soul want to go. When you have the feeling, then stay with it, and don't let anyone throw you off."*
>
> *Joseph Campbell,* ***The Power of Myth***

CHAPTER TWENTY FOUR

IN EARLY JUNE, Victor gave me an extraordinary gift. He asked me to accompany him to Seattle for the American Holistic Medical Association Conference. The gathering was held in a facility in the hills outside of Seattle, and for four days I was immersed in the atmosphere and energy of a remarkable group of men and women.

There were lectures, classes, demonstrations, and products. The days were filled with unparalleled learning and fine, quality speakers: Frank Hoffman, Alan Gaby, Dennis Jaffe, Bernie Siegel, Irving Oyle, Leonard Wisneski. Wisneski's talk about the immune and endocrine systems was incredible. He explained how science could actually measure the rise and fall of the body's lymph and other cells based on people's stress levels and the kind of thoughts they think.

I listened to the medical people and to the lecturers and I heard my own history explained. The high stress. The negative thoughts. All had suppressed my immune system and stimulated my endocrine system ... until it crashed, exhausted. I was convinced that I could build up my immune system and that handling stress was the key. My thoughts created my wellness or illness.

The second night at the conference was enlivened by the presence of a man in bed with my roommate. Then the morning was vitalized because my roommate inadvertently locked the dormitory room and left while I was down the hall in the shower. Dripping with water, I had to run into the dining room wrapped in a towel. Fortunately, I managed to quickly locate her and get the key, so a potentially awkward situation was nipped in the bud.

That day I met Marge, an RN from Montana, at lunch and later we sat in an allergy workshop and talked. I asked her questions about me and candida and MS and she whipped out her pendulum. The answers were "no-no." No candida problems and no MS. I was fascinated. Of course, we did the same thing at Victor's, but I'd never seen the pendulum before. Marge had picked up the magnetic vibrations from me through her hands.

She talked about castor oil for "Everything," and told me how to do castor oil packs on my back. How I wanted to go to Montana and take her classes. I was impressed that here was an RN teaching pendulums, castor oil, past lives, reflexology, etc. to nurses--and with the blessing of the medical establishment! It was thrilling and mind-boggling!

Another evening I sat next to an M.D. from Montreal who did magnetic healing, attended healing circles and was a psychic. I asked him to do a healing on me and he did. I kept wishing my mind would cease its inner chatter and stop trying so hard to "get it." I relaxed, but that's all I noticed.

On the third evening, I had an intriguing experience. Victor said he was going to test Wisneski. I asked Bob, the naturopathic student from Portland, to join us in Victor's room. The meeting turned into a powerful interplay and had, I'm sure, longer reaching, more profound effects than we could then know.

Victor had me lie down and he demonstrated the leg length testing. He told Wisneski how I was a tough case and how I still had leg problems, etc. So I popped in with my story, in brief.

Wisneski immediately said, "The spine chakra is blocked--not rising."

Then he looked at me sharply and asked, "Are you meditating?"

He had Victor ask, "Does Barbara have an energy blockage?"

"Yes," according to the legs.

"Does Barbara need to meditate and attend to that part of her?"

"Yes!"

Wisneski leaned over me and said, "I'm a doctor and I have a university degree and this and that and I know you're going to be all right," and he gave me a big hug.

Now things got even more exciting. Victor and Bob both took turns testing Wisneski, Victor with leg length and Bob with kinesiology. Their information matched and Wisneski was blown away. He'd never seen it done--which surprised me as he'd obviously been extremely open to "alternatives."

Victor and Bob checked Wisneski's adrenals and his foods and his yeast, then his mother who was ill, then some diabetic drugs and calcium theories that he was working on.

Victor asked, "Does Wisneski have psychic powers?"

"Yes."

Wisneski told us about the crystals he had used in the lecture that morning and how his entire lecture had unfolded as if someone else was talking through him. He felt that there'd been a special energy in the room that ebbed and flowed. Bob had been aware of it.

Wisneski was intensely moved by what he was learning. He saw all his activity of the last four months as preparation for this moment. I thought, *He has the credentials and he can take what he is learning back to the established medical arena.*

At the end of the session Wisneski turned to me and said, "There was something you had to hear from me tonight and there was something I had to hear from these two."

He also said, "That wasn't me who told you you'll be all right. That was your spiritual guide."

I knew he was right. I thought to myself, *I know I must get a meditation teacher. I have so much to learn.*

As Paul Brenner, the last lecturer spoke, I was aware that his message sounded much like that of Brugh Joy, and lo, a half hour into the talk he mentioned "My friend, Brugh Joy." I'd never heard of Dr. Brenner before, nor of his books. It was only after he'd been talking a while that I realized that he'd been right there at the conference all week. I'd seen the tall, average-acting and looking man here and there and never gave him a second thought. Now, as I listened, I realized that I'd spent the week in the presence of a very special, very remarkable person and it seemed astonishing that he'd never in the least attracted attention to himself.

He spoke with feeling and passion, without apology or fear, straight from the heart. He talked about the stages of the healer, and of his own progress from one stage to the other. As a doctor he'd had to learn, "I don't need the patient to get better in order to feel good about myself."

He told the audience of doctors, "If you are not there for the person, the patient opposite you, you are missing something. That person is there to teach you." He said, "Doctors are never taught about helplessness. They are taught: Hope. Hope is the killer. Accepting helplessness is learning to integrate."

His stories of his experiences with his patients, his lessons, his journey of awareness, were moving and powerful. As I listened, my eyes grew moist and I felt such an outpouring of my heart toward him and his spirit. By the end of the lecture I noticed other wet faces in the audience. Suddenly, spontaneously, the M.D.'s, Ph.D.'s, psychologists and nurses began singing *Let There Be Peace On Earth*, and the entire lecture hall resounded with the voices.

As Victor and I drove home from the conference I was pondering the question: *Where do I fit in?* I felt so drawn toward wanting to serve, felt that there was more for me than giving people programs or filling pill bottles at the Whole Health Center. That somehow I had more to offer and more to learn. I didn't yet see or know my vehicle. I felt the lack of specialized training. *Yet,* I told myself, *I must remember that I have wonderfully specialized knowledge based on my unique experiences. Somehow they are my credentials.*

Back in Portland, I was aware of another legacy of the conference; I knew that the spiritual path must be attended to with the same degree of energy, time and commitment as I had devoted to the nutritional path. I'd known this was true, but I had shoved it into the background, fitting it in only as it was convenient. As I told Wisneski, "It's easier to do externals."

I was sure now that the experience of the conference had come about in order to give me a signpost for my journey. The signs had been there all along. But I sped on by. This time I came right up against the signpost. In big block letters like a giant freeway sign it said: ATTEND TO MEDITATION.

I'd not known how to go about learning to meditate, so I had just muddled along in my own way as best I could. Now I must put out the energy for the search for a teacher, book, some kind of help, and prepare to make a commitment. No more procrastinating. *Do it Now!* The spiritual journey, which had begun three years before, was now in full swing. It was time for me to acknowledge it.

> *"The future enters into us, in order to transform itself in us, long before it happens."*
>
> *Rainer Maria Rilke*

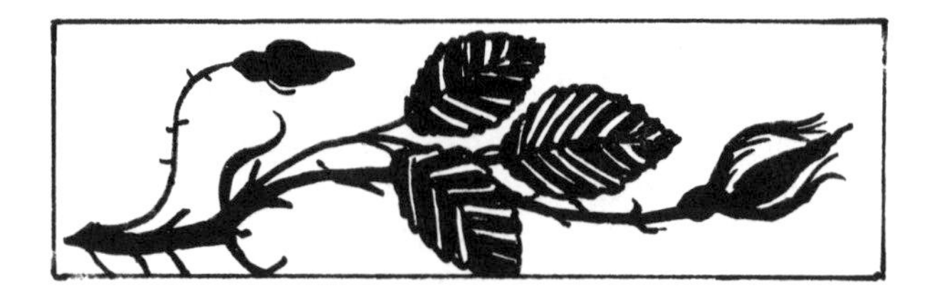

PART IV

THE PROCESS OF BECOMING

I can't understand why people aren't just dying to learn, why it isn't the greatest adventure in the world--because it's the process of becoming. Every time we learn something new, we become something new.

Leo Buscaglia, ***Living, Loving, and Learning***

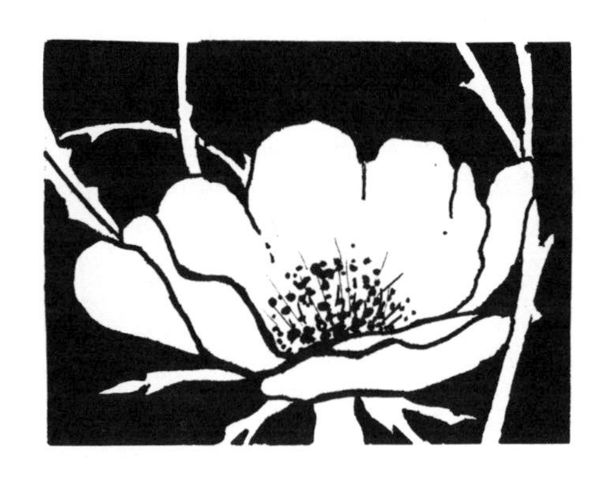

CHAPTER TWENTY-FIVE

NUTRITION BOOKS, BILLS and letters collected in unread, undone piles while I immersed myself in Catherine Ponder's *The Dynamic Laws of Healing*. I was consumed by the need to make some kind of spiritual adaptation. I felt that I was undergoing an internal gear-shifting, a response to the changes that had been going on, that were here now, and which were unfolding. They were not visible at the surface level. My life continued with "normalcy." But the underlying movements were grinding like the Pacific plates beneath the continent.

Interestingly, at this time, I discovered Catherine Ponder's term *chemicalization*. It referred to the wrenching, cleansing, purging process that takes place once a person starts on a positive path. After treading a long while on a negative path, then shifting to a different, uplifting, positive one, what could happen was that the body circumstances wouldn't readily adjust. The old entrenched thought processes couldn't let go without a fight. Therefore a chemical change was literally taking place in the thoughts and feelings, and it was reflected in the body or the prosperity or in other conditions.

This concept perfectly described what had been going on since the MS hit. In my case, illness was the crisis that instigated the first tentative steps toward changing my thinking. Once started, it had brought on one gear-grating, lurching process after another.

Listening to my Eileen Caddy tape, the repeated message was that I must hand my *all* over to God, or to WHATEVER, as Frances Horn put it. That I must trust completely. Despite longing for a spiritual balance, I hadn't taken the steps in that direction ... except as I could fit it into my schedule. Now I had to fit my schedule around my spiritual life. *The "how" will be shown to me,* I reassured myself. *The lesson is about attending to that part of me even when chaos, pressure, clutter and distractions surround me.*

It was also--ego. I'd been hung up in the ego and its goals in relation to my spirituality and to my desire for "credentials." I wanted the "M.A.," the "N.D.," the "N.C.," the "M.D."--whatever, so that I could have credibility--power, authority--externally conferred; so that I could impress people with my credentials and through that gain their respect and attention and thus "help" them.

Now, however, I had no doubt that the power to serve was inherent. I was currently, and knew that I would continue to be, functioning in *some* field. It would come not from degrees and letters, but from opening up my heart and letting go of the ego. I knew why I had been so intently drawn to Dr. Paul Brenner. The man was seemingly without ego. He didn't need the credentials and the titles. It was his experience and his open sharing that gave him his power. (Did we, though, listen more attentively because of the credentialed place from which he spoke?)

Suddenly, for a moment, fear completely dissolved. I *knew* that I could be all I desired, could have the spiritual peace I craved, could affect people positively--*when I was without ego.* It seemed so simple and so desirable to let go of the ego. Why on earth would I want to hang on to it? How wonderful it would be to lead my life without needing to impress people or gain their approval, without fear of hurting or intimidating them. Without ego so much was possible. Peace was possible.

A two-fold pattern was evolving, one that would take me a long time to transcend--and one on which I am still working. The body acted as the instrument for grabbing my attention. The more insistent it became, and the more frustrated and helpless I felt to remedy it, the more I became aware that there was only *one* resolution: to find peace within--in God, Self, higher power, WHATEVER.

It was also as if the body were the mirror reflecting the inner adjustments. The more that was shifting internally, the more I could expect physical discomfort--especially when I couldn't or wouldn't honor the inner readjustment. The changing consciousness inside me demanded that I keep up with it, but often I refused or simply felt helpless to do so.

One afternoon in late May, Bob, the Naturopathic student, dropped by The Whole Health Center and examined me. He said, "Your body is screaming for nutrients. How is your digestion?"

"Terrible."

"You're right," he said.

I was stunned as he rattled off all the body systems that were askew ... a lot of problems stemming from malabsorbtion.

"Your colon seems good, and that interests me," he said.

Although he was a doctor, I still laughed inwardly at that comment coming to me from a young man.

Discouragement settled like a shroud as he ticked off the list of problems to be handled. He tried to cheer me by saying, "Keep in mind, that you've come a long way."

I knew that was true. But my fears about MS and relapses and deterioration surfaced. Could I maintain a steady improvement? Was the damage so permanent that there was a limit to how well I would be? *NO! I know that's not true even as I think it.*

"The human body tends to move in the direction of its expectations."

Norman Cousins, ***The Healing Heart***

CHAPTER TWENTY-SIX

IT WAS THE first Saturday in June--the day of the firewalk. I spent the morning checking off my various chores and was fascinated watching my reactions. Amazingly, there was no nervousness. No fears one way or the other. I perambulated easily through my day totally accepting of whatever path I might choose--to walk or not.

At four o'clock I arrived at Steve Hillenger's house. From there the group of 17 shuttled out to the Helvetia countryside. Steve had us gather on a grassy riverbank down the hill from a private home. He instructed us to carefully build a massive pile out of the logs he had brought. They were set alight and huge, red flames raged up, forcing us to stand well back from the heat. While the fire burned itself down during the next couple of hours, Steve guided us through several processes. Some were "trust walks" (allowing ourselves to be led, eyes closed, by another person) and "trust falls" (falling backward off a table into the arms of six people).

As we shared our fears and our reasons for being there, I expressed my fear of sabotaging my walk. Of gearing up to walk on the coals, and *doing* it, and then halfway through deciding that this couldn't *really* be me, that it was too impossible. Thus I'd undermine myself--I'd not be able to follow through and I'd get burned.

"Sabotage" struck chords for me. I had sabotaged countless areas of my life. I thought negatively and sabotaged my business. I sabotaged my well-being and activity level by not sleeping. My interactions and contributions were sabotaged by being "ill." I allowed the food I ate to sabotage my body. I sabotaged my loving relationships by not being able to sleep with my partner. I disbelieved my own abilities and hence didn't manifest them. As I talked to the group, I realized, *It hasn't been my* ***body*** *that sabotaged me. It has been* ***me*** *that sabotaged my body and, through that, myself.*

That night I knew that I could let go of the sabotage. I allowed myself to embrace it as a tool, as a technique that had served its purpose in other times. How had it served me? It kept me from appearing too confident. Kept me meeting others' approval. Kept me from being "different," i.e. from being powerful and resourceful, which might have been intimidating both for myself as well as others. I began to see that walking through the fire would be a way to kiss sabotage goodbye. *I no longer need you.* The question of walking or not dissolved. It was just when--and how.

I was content to let others lead, knowing I'd walk when it was time. Secretly, I wanted to check their feet for burns. I didn't, though, as everyone simply walked across the ten foot expanse of coals and returned to their place in the circle as if nothing at all had happened to their feet.

When I moved into position, heart thumping and legs shaking with the enormity of the moment, I still didn't know if I would walk, even though I felt very trusting and certain that I was ready. The glowing coals shimmered like sunny water. I waded across. There was a slight hot feeling, as of walking across hot pavement on a July day. At the other side of the coals I let out a shout and jumped onto Steve with a bear hug just after he poured water over my feet. (He always washed any clinging coals from our feet, since once we'd stepped from the fire we returned to a different consciousness and might be burned.)

I wanted to walk a second time--to confirm that I'd really done it, and to see if I could still do it *and* just because I wanted to. This time the coals seemed hotter, but not much. The sensation was as if I'd just dashed through a wide creek of ice water.

We finished as a group, holding hands and walking single file through the fire.

When Steve suggested the group walk, I asked, "What happens if one of us drops out?"

He answered, "You have to decide now ..."

So I decided.

When we had discussed our fears prior to the walking, Steve had told us, "Your body will do what is right to handle the fire. Your mind will do what is right. Your spirit will do what is right."

Throughout the evening, I remembered that and believed it. When I got home at one in the morning, I believed it even more as I took off my shoes to look at my feet in the light. The soles looked as if they'd been in my shoes all the time--except for being rather dirty. Simply nothing to show that I'd just walked four times across red hot coals. Half of me was amazed; half of me said, *Of course.*

After the walk, our group filed inside the host's house for a snack. Looking at the repast, foods I'd normally forego because of their yeast or wheat or sugar, or other ingredients, I decided that I was no longer going to let food undermine me. So I simply ate what I wanted. There was no head reaction.

The next morning I was compelled to check my feet again. No sign of my walk across coals. It seemed incomprehensible that there wasn't even some little blackening, *something* to show what happened. Steve had told us, "Some people need proof of their accomplishment and they manifest it in blisters." I guessed that for me the proof was inside.

> *"Indeed, what is there that does not appear marvellous when it comes to our knowledge for the first time? How many things, too, are looked upon as quite impossible until they have been actually effected?"*
>
> *Pliny the Elder,* ***Natural History, Book VII, Sect. 6***

Karl arrived in the late afternoon. I told him about my firewalking and was quite surprised at how he needed to be defensive about his beliefs about reality. He couldn't allow that the coals had been "really hot." They had to be "cold"--say--300 degrees. It was too much for him to comprehend that ordinary people like myself could walk over 1200 degree coals and not get burned. He said he'd attend next time and bring his pyrometer and test the temperature.

Did *I* become defensive? As if he would undermine my experience? The experience was mine, not his, and I couldn't be responsible or concerned for his lack of believing.

We made love and then drove over to the Washington Square water slide. Ten times I scaled the steep stairs, with only a little oddness in the legs. I took it slowly, and the last two climbs Karl piggybacked me up, simply because it was quicker and easier. The slides were fun. How appropriate to have a peak time in my life like walking on coals and to punctuate it with a wonderfully frivolous play-time experience, almost equally as foreign to me, as water sliding. Another first followed. We played video games. I didn't need to do that again.

At the end of the day we kissed goodbye. I wouldn't be seeing Karl for another two weeks, which was okay. I turned to my meditation book and renewed my efforts to achieve a written description for my goal. It was: *To live in awareness of the God that is within me, and to recognize that the "I" in me is God. To continually be still and drop the ego so that I can be a vessel through which God, "I," or* ***IT****, flows to all those I meet.*

At the same time as I stepped into new territory via the firewalk process, I was proceeding into new turf in the form of meditation. I'd found a used book which seemed "right on" for me. The author explained that it was okay to meditate for just two or three minutes if that was what felt best. The way to spiritual growth was to read and study spiritual writings and teachings, to be around spiritually oriented people, and to practice being still. This groundwork, which was laid out in simple steps, seemed so much more easy and feasible for me than other teachings I had encountered which directed, "Now go sit and clear your mind of chatter."

Ironically, I didn't bother to note in my journals the title of that particular book. The message found in the books by that author would become the foundation upon which my future learning would rest. It wasn't until several months later, in the midst of my darkest, most hopeless period, that I would discover how profoundly these teachings would affect my life. The book, which I found in the secondhand book store, was *The Art of Meditation* by Joel Goldsmith.

CHAPTER TWENTY-SEVEN

I ENTERED THE PES (Personal Effectiveness Seminar) primed for change--eager to discover the gold beneath the dross--and ready to put to rest the detrimental beliefs, issues, habits, and behaviors that dominated me. I viewed the seminar as a construction site in which to chip away at old dead layers, and as a safe place in which to construct the new, strange, replacement behavior--a place in which to practice the art of becoming ME. Today, I also realize that something in me knew that I must gain independence, strength, and trust in myself outwardly before I could honor and trust the inner demands. So much exploded out of the PES and the seminars that followed. It is impossible to share more than tiny glimmerings of the light that illuminated the experience.

FROM MY SEMINAR NOTEBOOK:

Day One

MY PURPOSE IN BEING HERE

My purpose in being here is to open to those areas of my being which have been shut down or ignored. It is to grow in self-awareness and self-trust; to expand my love, compassion and understanding, both of myself and others; to break through old habits, limiting beliefs and sabotage behavior; to gain clarity on how I can create what I want; to strengthen my commitment to being and acting as I want to be: balanced.

AREAS WHERE I AM SETTLING FOR THINGS IN MY LIFE
1. Less income than I need from work.
2. Family relationship is reactive.
3. Health--still eat compulsively.
4. Health--settle for status quo instead of taking care of myself as I can.
5. Relationship--settle for approval rather than risking disapproval.
6. Settle for less spiritual time, study and commitment than I want.

Day Two

Last night we were told to go home and dream about our purpose in PES. I dreamed that there was chaos and confusion all around Victor and me. I sit him down and talk to him about how I can still live in Santa Cruz and commute and continue to work for him. There's a wedding party in a house and a sleeping child outside---whom we awaken.

Does this mean that I can work for Victor part time? That I can be in my own world (i.e. Santa Cruz) and commute into Victor's world --say three days a week? I only pass through the wedding party--am no part of it. Get rid of all the wedding flower stuff? The sleeping child is awakened by me and by the chatter of the other people. *Am I the sleeping child*?

So--is the purpose of PES to discover how I can have my home--inner life--complete, and still manage a career?

Present Day: Looking back, I'm struck by how profoundly the subconscious spoke to me in that dream. In the ensuing months and years, identifying, expressing, and sustaining that child was to become a major theme.

MY FIVE FAVORITE AVOIDANCE MECHANISMS
1. eating
2 organizing/busy
3. reading
4. being "nice"
5. walk away

MY TWO FAVORITE AVOIDANCE ROLES

1. Approval-Suck
2. Clown/Cute

HOW I GIVE AWAY POWER IN THE WORDS I USE

My language shoots holes in my personal power. If I have a pie and cut it into pieces, there would remain one tiny slice that represents personal power. All the other pieces would be given away by my use of terms such as:

But
should/could/would
try
I wish
I hope
I don't care
I can't
I don't know
They made me
I have to
If
I forgot
I apologize for existing

When I say, "I *have* to rest, work, write Christmas cards, change myself," choice is eliminated and I become a victim. When I substitute, "I *want* to," or "I *can*," I support myself acting from personal power, from choice.

Day Three

HOW I PLAY WIN/LOSE AND RIGHT/WRONG

More and more I am changing in those areas. Once I viewed myself as lesser if someone else was "greater," i.e. if they were right it somehow made me wrong. Or if they were winning then I saw myself as losing. Unbelievably, I would resent another's losing weight because I felt fatter by comparison. Instead of applauding another person's good luck, great job, weight loss or increased income, I saw it as confirmation of my bad luck, lesser job, fatness or lack of money. That mental comparing is still there but much less so.

I'm tuning in to the fact that only *I* win for Barbara. It is only when I act in accordance with what's so for *me* that I am right--or win. The only way I am able to truly judge that is by being very still and listening to the inner voice. I don't always hear it. It's easy to get caught up in busyness, distractions, desires and comparisons. But I know now that *I do not make myself right or make myself win if I make someone else lose or make them wrong.* It's very simple, yet very complicated to do in the face of the external bombardments.

THE EXPERIENCE CIRCLE

A realization dawned as a result of the Experience Circle process. The people in my group told me, "You have a big heart. You're very caring. You're compassionate. You take care of others, but you don't take care of yourself enough."

How could they pick up on that? What an awareness, because it is true. All the time with Jack, the feedback I got was, "You think only of yourself." I bought into that and beat myself up for it. I *did* take care of myself in trying to eat healthfully, in exercising, in working hard to keep up the money, in getting involved with Peter. But I really didn't take care of myself in the way that was necessary. I didn't love myself. I didn't give myself permission to be wrong, to be imperfect, to live with the disapproval of others.

Day Four

WHAT I WANT TO SAY TO DAD

You had to be right. As long as you were right it was okay for you even if it made the rest of us wrong. I sought recognition and love through gaining your approval. But you still didn't give of yourself deeply from love. As an adult, I can appreciate that you couldn't. That you loved your family through your own barriers and gave in the ways in which you were most comfortable--the college education, the trips abroad, the grand gesture. All the depth of emotion was ignored, and I missed that. I sought approval and what exhilaration swept me when I "did it right"--or did things you related to like hunting or shooting or riding horses.

You never gave me *you* and hence I could never give you me. I have only rare memories of being hugged by either you or Mom. I wanted the emotional depth and it was scrupulously ignored or squashed when I expressed it. In recent years I've taken risks and been vulnerable. In Santa Cruz this May, I still didn't get acknowledgement. But from your hospital bed you raised your right hand as I was leaving and it was like a salute.

WORKSHOP PROCESS

This afternoon we were taken through a long guided visualization as we lay in the dark on the floor. We were told to take whatever tools or materials were necessary and build a workshop or study where we could always go for peace, answers, retreat. After that we were to write one paragraph that expressed the *feelings* we had about that workshop. Then another paragraph that expressed its *traits.*

When we had completed that, we were told to go back and cross out the words "workshop" or "it" and replace them with "me," "I," or "myself." As I did so, I had a split second of recognition. The Ah Ha! experience:

My FEELINGS about ~~my workshop~~ myself are thankfulness that I finally have ~~it~~ me. Joy, exaltation, delight. I feel uplifted, closer to God. I feel spiritual about ~~it~~ me. Pleased and grateful to have ~~it~~ me. I feel drawn to ~~it~~ me. I feel safe in ~~it~~ me, uplifted, healed, close to heaven in ~~it~~ me. I feel trusting and filled with God's essence in ~~it~~ me.

The TRAITS of ~~my workshop~~ me are comfort, spacious, impeccably designed. ~~It is~~ I am a sanctuary, loaded with books and with the desks and chairs for study. ~~It is~~ I am a place with spiritual qualities, where I get close to God. ~~It is~~ I am warm and sunlit and high on a rim over a grand canyon. ~~It is~~ I am connected with God and with the sky. ~~It is~~ I am friendly, receiving, serene, secure, safe. ~~It has~~ I have meditation space. ~~It is~~ I am a healing space where peace and healing fill me.

Wow! Wow! Wow! Wow! Wow!

What an impactful experience. I read the words describing my study and when I replaced "study" and "it" with "me" and "I," I started to laugh in delight and discovery, and then the tears streamed down my face. Because the place that I described--the place that is the core in my heart's image--is just what I wanted it to be.

All this time I doubted, wasn't sure what was there. I've been seeking, seeking, seeking. Suddenly I'd described it all, and all that I'd described had come from nowhere else but inside of me. It came not at all from the outside. Discovery! Introduction! Embracing of me! And the heart's image is ALL, ALL that I want within me.

> *"There is a peaceful place inside*
> *that welcomes you.*
> *A space so safe, so still,*
> *that there is no forward or backward--*
> *only the eternal flow of Now.*
> *Enter this radiance*
> *where the truth of your being resides,*
> *and remember who you are."*
> *Rusty Birkus,* ***Appearances***

After the PES graduation and then dinner with Jan Paul, I drove home alone to stride on strong legs under the clear night sky and the crescent moon. Dim points of stars and the dark outlines of the trees soared against the fading horizon. I felt wonderfully full, serene, alive--glowing with the incredible movement of the previous five days. How far I had rocketed since Victor and candida and the Whole Health Center eons ago. I knew that I had moved into my spiritual center more than ever before. I was suffused in the awareness of being there. How right it felt.

I walked, quietly exhilarated, and just as I had in that first sundown on the Sydney Harbor Bridge so many years ago, I ran with arms outstretched. Just as then, I'd arrived, and now the adventure was really starting. At dinner Jan Paul had said, "The Whole Health Center is just temporary. I see you in teaching. It's not nutrition. It's teaching and it's spiritual." As I walked and ran with strength and sureness, I knew yet again that the process and purpose was for me to be strong and healed--for God's purpose--not for mine.

I thought, *I am a tool for God's manifestation--so that all who meet me meet God in me. Whatever work I do will require health and strength. I wonder if I'll be unable to access strength and wellness until I step beyond using them for my ego's satisfaction.*

> *"Desire to sow no seed for your own harvesting; desire only to sow that seed the fruit of which shall feed the world."*
> *Light on the Path, from* ***Hatha Yoga*** *by Kathleen Hitchcock*

CHAPTER TWENTY-EIGHT

TWO WEEKS AFTER the PES, my body was giving me lots of messages. I didn't like them. *How*, I wondered, *could I go through a growth experience such as the PES and still have a screwed up body*? I had bought a tape of Dr. Irving Oyle's, which linked disease with the images that we carry within ourselves. As I listened to the tape, I asked myself, *What image does* ***dis****ease give me? What purpose does it serve? What is the buttock pain telling me?*

I can't lie down. I can't sit down. ***Get off my butt!***

What is the image of the weak legs?

Stop moving. Slow down. Stop carrying your own weight. Your legs can't do it all. Come to rest.

What is the image of the indigestion?

I can't digest too much at once. Fill myself in small, frequent amounts so that it can be assimilated and understood.

I paid a visit to Dr. Khalsa. I was less than pleased to hear him tell me that candida was evident according to his testing. Back to the diet. In fact, he suggested that in order to rest the digestive system, I should go on a mono diet. I thought, *Ugh! How awful!* The truth was, though, that my body was crying for it. I hadn't wanted to take responsibility for such a strict move because I'd been so attached to my foods. "Attachment is the cause of all human suffering--" said who? Buddha?

Once I "digested" the idea of the mono diet and saw so many positives, I was actually eager to get on with it. Surprisingly I felt that I ***could*** do it. *If I walked over coals I sure as hell can eat rice* *and mung beans for a month.* What was a month in the time span of my life? The only negative was boredom. I had spent 40 years being stimulated by food. What a wonderfully important lesson. Could I not discover other stimulations? I truly wanted to do that.

> *"If you make a list of everything ... you prefer, that list would be the distance between you and the living truth. Because these are the places where you'll cling. You'll focus there instead of looking beyond."*
>
> *Stephen Levine, **Who Dies?***

Two weeks later, I was once again jetting south on a plane to Santa Cruz. Karl had just seen me off. What a different self-image I carried because of the time we'd spent together that morning. How unfamiliar it was to make love and then be chauffeured to the airport and kissed on my way by a man with whom I had a romantic involvement. The only other time that had happened was years ago in New Delhi with Edward. How I had ached with the leaving. How Edward and I had clung to the last hours and moments together, never guessing that he would be dead within the month.

This travelling felt so natural for me. I felt like I was regaining myself, my stride, my true way of being in the world--full of movement, relationships, fun, growth, learning, purpose. I looked down at the checkered landscape sprawling around Portland. A fine city to be from. Rich countryside, rolling hills, and fields surrounded the heart of the city. There loomed Mt. Hood, and Jefferson and the Three Sisters, and off in the distant clouds, St. Helens. Oregon below--beautiful, trim, verdant, straw-colored meadows and deep green colonies of trees, glints of buildings and ribbons of winding streams, so orderly, so tidy. I felt filled with aliveness, with exuberance for being there and for flying off to California, moving ahead joyfully in my life.

The trip had come up suddenly when Victor said, "Here's a conference you ought to go to," and shoved a flyer under my face. It was for the West Coast Dowsers Convention in Santa Cruz and was too made-to-order to pass up. Within the hour, I was booked for San Jose. Everything fell into place quickly and easily--the reduced fare, Victor paying my registration fee, the schedule. And I'd thought, "This is the way I live my life!"

We were flying over California--brown, dung-dry and grey. There stretched the Golden Gate Bridge. It hung suspended between grainy haze and grey-green water. Everything was harsh metallic glints and man-made greys. How long it had been since I had visited the City. Just flying over it, I was swept with memories. I felt so right--so me --flying there, moving, going and coming on trips and adventures, tapping into the places of my past as I moved forward with purpose.

> *"When I look back on my travels, I see an almost obsessive desire for experiences that would increase my self-awareness. I needed new experiences to keep shaking myself up."*
>
> *Michael Chrichton, **Travels***

From the moment I stepped out of the plane in San Jose, I was enveloped in a gay and sparkling adventure. At the airport I joined an assembly of dowser conference participants shuttling to Santa Cruz in four yellow cabs. I rode with Jim and Pat from Flagstaff and Wally from Puyallup, and I learned as I rode. Jim and Pat were both retired teachers and educational administrators and had been dowsing for several years. Pat read auras and performed healings.

I discovered that this was the pattern with those I met at the conference. Most were ordinary looking people who looked, talked and ate the traditional American way. Many of the men were overweight, the classic caricature of the American man with "Dunlop's Disease" (when de belly dun lop over de belt). They favored polyester shirts and the women wore floral moo moos. They had family picnics, and along the way they dowsed. Most of them were older people who had never heard of Brugh Joy or Stephen Halpern. But they had been swinging their rods and wires and pendulums without fanfare for years.

I quickly learned that there was much more to dowsing than I'd known. In fact I thought it was really misnamed. It should have been called "magnetics," or "energizing," or "divining," as it's known in Australia. Dowsing was certainly not reduced to simply searching for water sources. As I talked with dowsers and saw the list of conference speakers, I realized that what was called dowsing was really a form of energy conducting, and it could be directed into many different areas.

These traditional-looking, middle-class Americans were using forms of dowsing techniques that had been around for thousands of years--for healing, for reading auras, for veterinary medicine, for spiritual connections, for searching for archaeological sites, for planning where to build highways, buildings, roads, wells, for measuring the energy and healing qualities of gem stones, locating energy blockages in people or animals or places, locating gold or oil as well as water, for psychological counselling ... !

How I loved learning all this. How fortunate I was that Victor had wanted me to come. How perfect that I could attend the conference and visit my family at the same time.

The first evening, I attended the opening ceremony with Dick from Tucson---Dick, the 60-year-old wrangler in his cowboy boots and hat. He pulled out his pendulum and as the speakers talked, Dick picked up their energy by the degree of rotating that the pendulum exhibited. Handing me the pendulum, he instructed, "Concentrate on receiving the speaker's energies." The pendulum bobbed but the movement wasn't as pronounced for me as for Dick. When I concentrated on NO energy, then it stopped.

It was so easy being with these people. All were open and friendly and there was no sense of one trying to be more mystic than another. I liked the way we were simply given name tags with no titles strung after them. Only when a speaker was introduced did it come up that Mr. X was a NASA engineer, or Miss Y was a Ph.D., and so and so, who was talking about magnetic healing, was an M.D. How different from other conferences where people had had their letters and titles blazoned across their chests.

The afternoon of the second day, we beginners practiced our new dowsing skills in the redwood grove. Dick, my wrangler friend, took me and my new dowsing rods in hand--literally--and I was thrilled at the wire rod responses. Then a group of three men clustered around me, dowsing me with pendulums and bobbers or springs. Dick found a meridian to zap with his acupuncture zapper and some "hot spots" on my back in which to grind his finger into my flesh.

After dinner our hands were read in preparation for the upcoming hand class. The leader studied our "simian" lines. These lines are evident across the first third of the palm when the hand is partially bent. We were told that "simian" meant "monkey" and that a solid line meant the person had "simian hands," while a partial line meant one was a "partial simian." Only 10% of the general population, we were told, had simian hands, while at dowsers conventions the speaker found 70% simian hands. Downs Syndrome children had this type of hand, as did geniuses. Thus I had no idea how to respond when I was told that both my hands were simian.

Most of my days were spent with my swirl of men, especially Harold, the retired army colonel from Arkansas, and my friendly cohort, Dick. I enjoyed them and felt their affection for me. They both gave me zealous encouragement with my dowsing, looked after me in gentle, subtle ways and, beaming at my enthusiasm, patiently answered my questions. At meal times, one or the other would greet me in the cafeteria and invite me to a table with them. Together they helped me dowse for "noxious rays" on a map of my house. Harold offered to go digging at the crystal mines in Arkansas and promised to send me some crystals for the Whole Health Center.

Such a convergence of male energy surprised and, of course, delighted me. Men, mostly 60 or older, had clustered around me "like flies to fly paper," as my neighbor Ruth so graciously put it. I decided that it must be my new energy make-up that people were picking up on. As I integrated my various selves and as I discovered and accepted my spiritual self, perhaps I created a certain attracting energy.

> *"People, whose own self-respect immunizes them against resenting you for your self-love, will prefer you, seek you out. Why? Because people that accept themselves, are usually a pleasure to be with."*
>
> *Paraphrased from,* ***I Want to Change, But I Don't Know How***

As the conference drew to a close, so too, a cloud of loss closed around me. I was reluctant to see the high time cease, to stop the flow of the intense learning, to say farewell to the friendly people with whom I felt comfortable and who had so quickly become a part of each day. I was reluctant to stop the deluge of information, and yet I did need some time to practice and to absorb.

I said goodbye to my new friends and dedicated the remaining five days in Santa Cruz to interacting solely with my family. Each day I went alone, or with Mom or Sis, to the nursing home where my father was staying. In the course of that time, as I gently introduced new ideas, I saw the changes in Mom and Dad, the uplift in both of them.

Taking the initiative in guiding and helping my parents was both exhilarating and a stretch. In each approach that I tried, I had to put aside my fears of "doing it wrong" or being misunderstood. Although touching one another was something my family carefully skirted, I massaged Dad with total confidence, without shyness. I played my Eileen Caddy tape for him, sure of the need and of the right timing for it. I coaxed this man, who lay lethargic and hopeless, to squeeze his hands around an imaginary golf ball, and I showed Mom how to massage his feet. She readily leaped to try, finally having a sense of being able to do something. To my sister, who viewed new or different approaches with uncertainty, I gave love and respect, encouragement and praise. And, strangely, I found it easy--not fake or artificial.

I arranged with a therapist to give Dad a series of massages--the first he had ever had. I persuaded the holistic M.D., Dr. Houston, to agree to come on the case. Things fell into place. I felt effective and that I was making a real difference for Mom and Dad. With surprise, I realized that I, myself, was a vehicle for healing. Whether I "healed" through words, or cooking, or hypnosis, or with my hands, or by taking people to lunch, the vehicle was me.

Throughout the week I continued taking risks and trusting that the right thing would be said or done. As I left Santa Cruz, I felt a profound sense of satisfaction. And, I carried a deepening trust that whatever learning or training I needed would be put before me. As I became ready for the next step, it would be there.

> *"I think the meaning of our existence is not invented by ourselves, but rather detected."*
>
> *Viktor Frankl,* ***Man's Search for Meaning***

CHAPTER TENTY-NINE

NO SOONER HAD Karl delivered me home from the Portland airport than Eric Malin, the Dutch dowser whom I'd met in Santa Cruz, phoned. He was visiting Portland from his home in British Columbia. I invited him over, grateful for the chance for Karl to be exposed to some authentic dowsing.

Eric dowsed the yard and house until nearly midnight and then camped overnight in his van in the driveway. The next day I arrived home from work to find him and a trail of wood stakes and directional markers strewn around the lawns and the house. According to Eric's dowsing, the place was a stew of noxious rays. No wonder I'd had health problems. I tagged along behind Eric practicing with my dowsing rods, learning much from him, and relishing the thought of the spectacle that the two of us must have presented to the neighbors.

Two nights later, I attended the farewell dinner for the local macrobiotic teachers, Mark and Anna. Evidently I was looking as good as I felt because Anna, in her direct way said, "You look beautiful."

Later, as we parted she said, "It has been an enrichment knowing you. You're so eccentric."

I laughed, loving her guilelessness, and said, "Thank you. I'll take that as a compliment."

She quickly said, "I mean, we've met some eccentric people here in Portland and you're one of them."

I glibly responded, "Well, I'm working at it."

She answered me seriously, "I don't feel like you work at it. You just are."

I then proceeded to confirm her assessment of my eccentricity by telling her and Mark about my 29-year-old boy friend and about my "eccentric" evening the previous night dowsing my yard for noxious rays with a Dutch witcher. I drove home invigorated by the memory of Anna's words, and chuckling, *I'm already fulfilling my goal of living as if I'm 80.*

"You play first, last, and ultimately to an audience of one."
Read and Rusk, ***I Want to Change, But I Don't Know How***

Three days later, Eric was still camped in the driveway. Every night I returned home and he was busy dowsing. I went out to dinners or to classes or to swimming and then wanted only to come home and be alone. But no sooner did I settle down then Eric showed up to visit. Eric explained to me that by the time he was finished there would be forty 18" pieces of rebar driven into the lawn and garden. Supposedly they would deflect the rush of underground noxious rays that ran into and through the house. I was grateful to him for his generosity with his talents and because he was willing to drive the rebar in for me.

The day that Eric finally left Portland, Jack and I went out together. Over Chinese dinner we handled the divorce settlement. So easy. So simple. We talked about many other areas, especially spirituality.

As I told Jack about my new way of living he said, "Will you marry me someday?"

Although he said it in fun, I was touched by his sweetness. Later, when we parted, Jack said, "I hope the next one is as easy as this." He reminded me of how when we were dividing up the household stuff, we'd kept urging items on each other, and he'd said, "I'm so glad I married you. You're so easy to divorce."

I returned home radiant with pleasure in the evening, aware of the integrity and friendship Jack and I had accessed as we'd both grown in the last years. We both came from a place of loving and of only wanting the best for the other. It *was* easy.

It amazed me that I had time for dowsing or dinners or anything! The Whole Health Clinic demanded every ounce of my energy and time. Such a place it was! The days dashed along punctuated by deadlines and foul-ups, people phoning, interruptions, shipping orders, and catching up with Victor once he'd returned from a month in England. I dragged myself home at night, too tired to swim or to prepare food. My personal life languished on hold. I couldn't manage a spare hour for seeing Dr. Khalsa or Karl, for filling out the medical or insurance forms, for meditating ...

Victor reminded me of a child with a swarm of hornets following him around. There was a frenetic energy about him that seemed to hover between success and disaster. I saw the potentials for both. I believed the good outweighed the pitfalls, but his pitfalls tripped him up now and then. In our association these had been minor but, nevertheless, undermining. Since returning from England, he had acted very intense and irritable. I knew it was from lots of pressures, but it was difficult not to feel personally under attack.

During those summer weeks my energy dragged and my legs slugged. The work seemed offensive, the office torturously hot. There were no long periods of consistent attention on one project. The constant interruptions were the equivalent to having rifle shots snapping off around me every ten minutes. I was back in the Bloomers trap and I knew that something must be done.

The message from the Whole Health Center situation was that it was time to move on. To what? My task was to be still and to listen and be open to WHATEVER. *There are **no** accidents,* I told myself. *I'm being led and guided. My life is for joy--for bringing joy to others. I'm currently learning how to manifest that in the face of obstacles. Bless the gifts of these obstacles. I learn from them. Victor is a gift. Such lessons. Such an adventure I'm on. It's just like old travel days. I set out each morning and each week for certain points and as I achieve them, new destinations that I didn't dream existed open to me.*

> *"It is the direction of our progress that matters--not where we stand at present."*
>
> *N. Sri Ram, in Kathleen Hitchcock's* ***Hatha Yoga***

Diversion from my work problems arrived in the fashionably-clad form of my English friend, Judith, who lived in British Columbia. With her I could share raunchy, flip conversations, laughter, and my innermost questions. Typical was the evening we came home buzzy-headed at midnight after a fun, elegant evening on the town. The night had been a coming-out occasion for both of us. For me, it was celebrating the arrival that day of a check, my share of Dad's property sale. With the check came my opportunity to repay Judith for having bought my airline ticket to Vancouver four years earlier. The check was the long awaited passport out of penny pinching and hand-to-mouth economics. I had trusted that this day would eventually come, but had had no idea how long I'd have to wait or how big the check would be. It had seemed crass to ask Dad or to try to figure it out.

For six months I'd lived my life as if I was certain of this incoming windfall. It had been a scary thing to do--juggling payments, loading up the Visa--but now I applauded my decision. Because I survived. I flourished. I managed without having to give up certain priorities and necessities. Something had indeed looked after me.

Much remained unknown. What exactly would I be allowed to do with the money? Would I be able to keep most of it? Or would the government end up with half of it? Certainly there should be enough to pay off the doctors and credit cards and buy Jack out of the house. I might even be able to live for at least a year without having to work. I *knew* that the money was not there for me to be frivolous. It offered a platterful of opportunities. The challenge was in knowing how to use them.

During that festive night with Judith, money, for once, was no object. Decked out in our fancy outfits, we started with drinks and gay repartee at Atwater's on the 36th floor of the US Bank tower. I gave Judith the lion mug that she'd admired in the store earlier in the day and which I'd bought and snuck out of the shop with the clerk's help. Later at the Heathman, we each ate exactly what we wanted. Judith delicately nibbled pheasant in raspberry sauce and I feasted on giant, hand-sized prawns wrapped in bacon. (No MS diet here!) Judith chose a $25 bottle of French *pouilly foise*'--the most expensive wine I'd ever tasted.

Our conversation ebbed and flowed, full of Judith's droll witticisms--often at her own expense. What a mixture she was, this dear friend whom I first met in Bangkok, and then again, by coincidence, on a New Delhi street. She was at once so worldly and fashionable, and yet she was able to make fun of her vanity and behaviors. She quoted Shaw with her best Stratford-Upon-Avon British actress accent, and then punctuated it with the raunchy language of a trooper. Our exchange that night grew even livelier as we reached the end of the meal and the end of the wine bottle, which we couldn't finish. We both considered it a sign that we'd really *arrived*, that we were able to leave the remains without regret.

> *"I've got these friends I can count on,*
> *And they can love and let be,*
> *I've got these feet that can dance,*
> *Celebration of me!"*
> from, ***I'm Getting My Act Together and Taking It on the Road***

The week with Judith hurtled past like a comet, and once more I wrestled with questions about how I should proceed with my life. One Saturday as I worked in the yard, I used the time to grasp at and examine the shadows and glimmers of ideas and possibilities that danced into and out of my consciousness. I paused often to write--and process.

My morning thoughts started with the issue of the windfall of money. I was discovering that having the money clarified some matters and confused others. On the one hand, I wanted very much to earn my own way, to participate in people's lives, to do some purposeful work that was healing both for others and for myself. Certainly I could do that at the Whole Health Center. *The essence, however, of giving and healing has to come from within myself, no matter what I do or where I choose to work.*

On the other hand, if I handled the money wisely, I could literally do what I wanted. I could stop working entirely! I could bundle myself off to Australia and renew life and friendships there. I could travel to sacred sites, visit ashrams and meditation retreats. I could go to school full time. I could do nothing but attend workshops and seminars.

What an incredibly unique position. I could actually choose what direction I wanted my life to take! How frustrating that I didn't have enough sense of my purpose to be able to look at the options and simply know which was the one for me. If only I had some clearly defined goals and a strong sense of my burning desire, then wouldn't the decisions be instantaneous?

At midday I wrote some more. *The answer for my purpose is--as always--"go within." As usual, that is the only answer.* How ready I always was to remove myself from that course, busying and distracting myself with other things. Could I not accept, as I had during the winter, that I was still in a limbo, developing time? That it was not necessarily essential for me to *know* where I was going? That the key was to flow with my feelings?

Go for the growth, my feelings were saying--*whatever that may entail.* That had to be what the money was for. To enable me to pursue the path of growth and learning without the pressures and distractions of laboring flat-out five days a week. *By following my feelings,* I reassured myself, *I'm not heading down the path of ruin and irresponsibility. There* ***is*** *guidance in what I experience as my intuition. I need to learn to listen and to act in harmony with it.*

I'd been conditioned to believe that the only reality for being independent, successful and effective in the world was to work hard and long, push, be exhausted. I was opening to another reality, to accepting that for some reason ***my*** path might be otherwise. I was being offered the choice. I could move off my past position or I could continue to cling to my familiar concepts of how I gained approval, self-esteem and identity.

As the day and my pondering progressed, I edged closer to a sense of how to proceed. There was less equivocation. I became certain that my direction lay in stepping back from the long hours at the Whole Health Center and to directing my time toward self-exploration, spiritual learning, and personal growth. The goal grew clear. *I must do all I can to gain insight and to become a person who can be valuable in the personal transformation field.* People around me were doing so, and with no more talent or experience than I had. All I needed to do was to focus, to streamline, to move forward decisively.

I wrote: *I believe I can be effective without a degree. I do need the knowledge and skills, but I can pick those up without going the traditional route. I'll learn much more too.* People--Karl--were all essential in this process. The dialogue with him and others gave me the chance to practice expressing myself clearly in risky topics and to not cop out by using avoidance mechanisms like being lazy, vague or cute.

As sundown shadows streaked orange across the lawn and garden, I sat on my front steps feeling relaxed and purged. How important this day had been. A day without obligation, free to soar and roam in my thoughts and in my activities. I had savored the brilliant blue sky and the healing warmth of the sun. I loved the physical activity and the sense of accomplishment as I looked at the cleaned up yard and the mountainous pile of brush and limbs heaped on the lawn.

I felt comfortable with this process of work and exploration, of rest and writing. It had brought my brain to clarity. There had been no instantaneous flash, no sudden "ah-ha!" Rather, the awareness of my goals, of my purpose, of the path to be taken had gradually germinated and sprouted inside of me. There was no clear-cut line of Before-Decision and After. There was no Moment of Decision. Only a moving forward with ever increasing assurance of the rightness of that direction.

I thought, *I've come through this day to an embarkation upon the next segment of my journey.* How grateful I was for the calm and freedom, for the time to delve within where I could let the answers percolate up to my consciousness.

What a lesson. What a process. I must always remember that it is available. ***When I must make some sort of decision, I give myself a quiet day****, one in which there are no people, no projects, no deadlines or distractions. I write, I sit quietly. I move through the yard in perfect peace. As I move through the day in this way, I open up to what the voice within is saying.* I even forewent the pleasures of the swimming pool. It was so important to be without distraction. I did no letter writing, no bill paying. Yet the enormity of what had been accomplished filled me. I was wonderfully calm, at peace, perfectly positioned for my forward movement.

I embrace this entry! It so clearly expresses what was to become the pattern for how guidance operates in my being--if I will but let it. Foolish woman that I am, after seeing it work, I still forget. I still want immediate, cymbal flashing, explicit instructions. This entry reminds me--so beautifully--that if I turn the process over to inner workings, go about my business in a non-distracted way, the insights and guidance will come.

"The quieter you become the more you can hear."

Baba Ram Das, in Jon Winokur's ***Zen To Go***

CHAPTER THIRTY

THE EVENING AFTER my day of gardening, writing and processing, I attended Jack's PES graduation. It turned out to be open, easy and beautiful. When I entered the training room, Jack tearfully embraced me saying, "I love you!" and "You couldn't have given me a better gift!" I was relieved after my qualms about how he would handle going through the seminar at the same time as Karl. After talking with Jack, I then moved on to Karl and hugged and greeted him. Jack came over and hugged us saying, "I love you both," and to me, "I'm so pleased and happy for you because you've found a friend like Karl. I've seen these last few days what a wonderful, sweet person he is."

Wow! How we've both changed, I thought. I loved Jack for his openness, for traveling through the seminar, and for accepting Karl and me for who we were.

Three days later Karl and I left for Eugene and for the Cross Over Seminar. Cross Over was the second-level seminar that followed the PES. It was like hopping on to a roaring train after being on a motorcycle. Whereas PES opened participants to their hidden magnificence, Cross Over revealed their games and traps, the places in their personalities that tripped them up. I was in for an intense, rip-roaring ride. It was difficult, devastating, and, ultimately, powerfully releasing. The destination was definitely worth the journey.

FROM MY SEMINAR NOTEBOOK:

Morning of Day One

The pulsating of my body, the tension, the tightness in my stomach, the shortness of breath, the deep exhaustive sighs, all express the stretching that is underway here. I'm anxious about being told what I project to others--the things about me that don't work for them. I fear discovering the truth of all the trips, behaviors, games and numbers and illusions that I am running. Total exposure. Yet I anticipate and glory in it for *knowing the truth shall make me free*. It is the only way to self-knowledge and self-growth.

I'm split, at once fearing the learning, but wanting it too, because it will tell me what I am and what I do--both to myself and to others. I can choose to use this information as a tool for growth and change. Acknowledge myself for being willing to do this, to subject myself to painful self-learning.

I also dread telling Karl and the others the things I perceive in them that don't work for me. I might be wrong, might hurt them, they might reject me. I'm breathless, keyed up like the moments prior to shooting a major rapid.

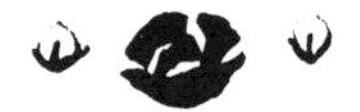

I'm wounded, pissed, numb, shut down, want to sleep, tired, concerned that I may not be letting in the learning. What horrible things to be told about myself. I wonder if I dare share myself again. I'm hurt that people think I use the hearing loss as a crutch. When I asked them to speak up I came across rude and see it now. After a lifetime of isolation and missing out because I *wouldn't* ask for people to speak up, I now ask for what I need and I screw it up. It's the *way* in which I ask.

I'm seen as spoiled, selfish, brattish, expecting my way. I feel tremendous self-loathing. How can anybody like or love me? How can a relationship possibly survive such revelations? I want to explain about the hearing disability. The perception by others is so distorted. Yet it must be there or else they wouldn't perceive it.

I don't want to share anymore, because I'm told that no one wants to hear me, that I'm explaining empty, pointless things. Throughout the process I was so focused on me, on formulating my own answers to questions, that I couldn't focus on the others.

I'm sure the relationship with Karl is dead, dead, dead. Maybe it never was alive. He's seen me revealed.

"Risk taking is the major part of the "cure" so don't hope that somehow you'll be able to avoid it."

*Read and Rusk, **I Want to Change, But I Don't Know How***

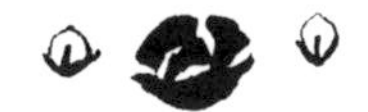

Mid-Afternoon of Day One

We are told to write about What Is My Greatest Emotional Pain? It comes from realizing that I am empty. That there *is* no emotion. That I've been shut down for so long. The pain is slow in emerging. I can't at first pinpoint it or feel it. Of course there have been painful experiences, but I can't recapture the *feeling*. There is no dramatic loss or incident about which to tell a story as others do.

Then I begin to access the hopelessness and sadness about the times when I've felt left out, apart, lonely. I grow sadder as I realize how out of touch I've been with those feelings. Rick, our small-group leader says, "It's been a long time since you've allowed those feelings to surface. It takes a while for you to get in touch with them." First, I felt guilty because I have no deep emotional pain such as others express. Then the sadness spills over because I see and feel that I am a dried-up shell.

Finally, the pain surfaces and I can hardly contain it. The truth is awful. I am dry, dead. I'm filled with self-hate and self-loathing and disgust. The pain is in having been so *un*feeling--in not having been there for myself or others.

"The pain can purify the mind and body; it burns out many obstructions."

*Dan Millman, **Way of the Peaceful Warrior***

Day Two

Awoke refreshed and alert. A shower revives--literally washing away the old stuff, the toxins. I'm quite calm and okay and ready to forgive myself for being the way I've been. I was that way and behaved as I did because I was using my best information and tools at the time. I am accountable for those choices and I can now choose to act differently. I can take the valuable information and know that I don't have to be that way again.

I don't have to call myself a bad person, because these were only outer manifestations, images. Yesterday I hated and loathed the person that was shown to me. Today I want to negotiate the next steps to forgive that person, to say goodbye to ugliness, and not dwell on it. I'm ready to take the tools that are offered and to learn how to change those unrewarding ways--to let go of the old and move on. I don't have to maintain myself as I was. Knowing the truth at last, I *can* move on.

Today I'm ready to share, eager to express the catharsis that is taking place. I let go of fear of being dull or dry or wrong or judged.

Day Three

Yesterday afternoon we discussed the different games that people run. The processes of the last three days have certainly revealed mine to me. Therefore, I found last night's homework, to write about "How I Run My Favorite Game," easy. The words came tumbling out almost ready-made, even though it was two o'clock in the morning.

THE AVOID-DANCE

or

Nine Ways to Avoid Self-Disclosure and Stay Approved Of

by

Able Side Stepper

Do you want to keep loving, bonding, and connection out of your life? Do you desire to keep people as separate from you as possible? If so, there are several handy methods available. These avoidance tactics are best employed by those who want to insulate themselves and remain out of touch with their true feelings.

It is important to practice and perfect these mechanisms, since doing them inelegantly can trip you up. The goal is certainly *not* to end up looking foolish. At least, though, as an insulated person, you won't have to worry about having close friends around you to see you being a fool. I speak from vast experience, having learned the Avoid-Dance early. Here are some of my favorite ways to side-step issues:

1. Change the subject. As soon as your friend or partner starts to push your buttons you can mention that the garbage man is coming tomorrow and you wonder if you should put out one can or two.

2. Get tired. It's very hard to focus on intimate, risky subjects if you're feeling sleepy. I caution you that this works best if it's late. Sometimes it's hard to get people to buy into it if it's early in the morning.

3. Get muddled. This is perfect for those times when you are already confused to begin with. If you don't know what to say anyway, you might as well say what you're not saying by using run-on, backwards, roundabout, fragmented sentences. This serves not only to keep you in confusion, but to bring your partner into it as well.

4. Get flirty or cute. Not to be used at executive conference meetings. This is best employed in those shaky moments when a mate puts you on the spot. It can be fun and distracting and serves very well to diffuse any chance that you might communicate intimately and honestly.

5. Do distracting physical things. Also best done with a partner or mate, rather than business associates. These could include sucking his/her toes, faking a charley horse or sticking your fingers in their ears.

6. Physically leave the area. This adequately interrupts the communication flow before it can get too deep. Going to the bathroom is a tactic I frequently use. Caution: this one can be annoying to your mate if the conversation is taking place in the car on a freeway. At-home disruptions that are ideal for Woo-Woos include exiting to turn on the water purifier or having to rinse your bean sprouts.

7. Suggest going to eat something. This is a favorite avoidance device and one that is usually well received both by mates and by the general public.

8. Explain. This can be a sure-fire way to avoid honest communication. It's great for displaying how many view points you hold or how much you learned at the last personal growth seminar. Of course, the more you do it the less capable you are of recognizing where the true bones of the matter are, so this technique really builds on itself. It can take hours, too, and I find it effective with self-righteous folks because they tend to demand a lot of justifications.

9. Brain Games. This is similar to explaining, and it's wonderfully useful when you're with another brain-bound person since they always rise to the bait. If you turn the conversation into analyzing, you can be pretty certain that you'll never have to worry about dealing with feelings.

You will find these techniques useful in keeping your relationships at a distance. I am available for consultation on any and all of these mechanisms and would profoundly encourage you to practice them diligently in order to become a master of them as I have.

What a delightful, humorous way to be revealed to myself. I feel silly seeing the methods I've used to avoid issues. Last night's conflict with Karl was such a gift for both of us. In the course of it, I saw exactly how I avoided the issue, how I expressed myself in a scattered, non-centered way. It became so easy to write my Avoid-Dance statement after I'd seen my game so clearly. I think I'm being nice to others *and* being safe and protecting myself. Instead, I create extremely negative responses and I shut people away and turn them off.

Today I went to Karl and said the truth--with everything to the point. The relationship *is* important to me. I *am* worried about it. I felt cleaned up, lighter, doing things completely differently. What an incredible gift. Pare down the words! Speak only about the core. Dispense with explanation.

SEXUAL BARRIERS

I CREATE SEXUAL BARRIERS BY:

1. Being under time pressure.

2. Getting very tired: by not sleeping well and thereby lacking the energy to have sex energetically or long or often.

3. Overeating: by getting too full and then not feeling comfortable enough to have sex. I also feel unattractive when I'm full or bloated and don't want my partner to see me that way.

4. Setting up rules and limits verbally or by not responding physically.

5. Avoiding: by silence, or by diffusing difficult questions.

6. Not asking for what I want.

7. Not being exploratory or inquisitive.

8. Being embarrassed, and thus holding back.

These behaviors are barriers whose goals are to keep me from losing face and from looking like a nerd.

I CREATE SENSUAL BARRIERS BY:

1. Choosing not to wear sensual underwear or night clothes even though I have them available.

2. Choosing clothes that are non-revealing, or selected for comfort as opposed to sensuality.

3. My bedroom is a sensual barrier. It could be tidier and could have decor that is more sensual, like photos or mirrors. I don't employ candlelight or music even though it would be easy to do so.

4. I do not introduce attire such as garter belts or stockings which might enhance or expand the quality of sensuality.

5. I limit my expression of wishes or desires. Fear of losing face, i.e. I could ask a partner to slow down the process, but I don't often do that. I don't interrupt my partner's flow or methods. Fear of doing it wrong.

6. Oil is available and I forget about it.

Day Four

Bev, our masterful trainer, gives me two tasks. The first is: be honest, share my feelings, be connected with heart and head. Do this with Karl--in front of the whole group. Practice self-disclosure. That is the route I must learn if I'm to have connection and love in my life. To practice on Karl is to learn how to be sharing, disclosing,

bonded--with others, with family, with friends, with men, Victor ...
The second task is: be a little girl--in front of the group.

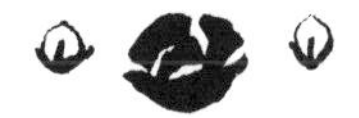

Karl and I face each other in two swivel chairs. The group sits in a horseshoe in front of us. Taking a deep breath, I plunge in.

"Karl," I say, "I've been happy to feel girlish and excited sexually with you. You've helped push me, in a fun way, out of my comfort zone. Even the head stuff, the verbal fencing and long talks, have been fun. I've learned to express passion and take pleasure in having fun with sex.

"But I've also felt judged by you. I feel that you have no idea of my real capabilities, that you discount me beyond the sexual, light, frivolous roles I've played with you.

"Sometimes you seem like a little boy, pouting and spoiled. In many ways I feel so much stronger--simply from the experience of life. Sometimes I wish you'd just get on with your life, instead of living with your parents and dragging around. I like the sex, but I'm unhappy with your distancing and the lack of loyalty. I don't think I can go on with a relationship in which there is no depth of commitment."

Karl seems to take it all well. He sits quietly, an almost quizzical expression on his face. He is not expected to respond in this process. But at the end, there are tears in his eyes as he says, "Thank you. I appreciate your honesty. And I do love you."

Whew! I'm so drained I can barely rise from the chair. But my second act must follow. The chairs and Karl are removed and I become a little girl. The nervousness quickly drops away as I dive in--chattering and babbling, crawling and dancing, coloring a book, seeing a caterpillar, talking to "Mommy," and pointing at the "dogs" mating on the lawn. At this point Bev stops me, saying, "Great, Barbara. You've got the point."

Checking in on my feelings now I'm cleansed, light, released. With Karl, I feel more connected even though I know we're parting. I feel clean with the honesty. The secret is to stay connected. Stop going to my head to think or plan about how to talk to Karl from my feelings. All I have to do is check into the little girl. She lives only in the moment. She doesn't plan "how" to do something. She embodies my new commitment and my lesson: remember the little girl. She is delight, love, honest communication, and her head is always connected with her heart. So easy. Slow down. Go to my feelings.

Evening of Day Four

As the day progresses, I'm really getting connected, like the little girl, completely, in the moment, with life's surprises and delights. I do not leave life--the moment--travelling to my head to plan and scheme so as to be ready for the next life situation that I'm anticipating. Be here now. The only situation I need to plan for is the one I'm in right now. Keep remembering and reconnecting with the little girl--with the joy and wonder and delight of each successive moment.

> *"Did you have a happy childhood?" is a false question. As a child I did not know what happiness was, and whether I was happy or not. I was too busy being."*
>
> *Alistair Reid, in Jon Winokur's* ***Zen To Go***

All at once, I remember my dream on the first night of PES back in June. There was a sleeping child who was awakened. I'm awed to realize how my subconscious spoke to me then and how now, two months later, the meaning is percolating into my consciousness.

Day Five

AFTER REBIRTHING PROCESS

We lay on the floor tucked in with blankets and pillows.

I'm taking deep breaths, modifying my breathing. I can't believe I'm not hyperventilating.

My ears seem plugged up.

My left leg is icy cold, numbish.

My hands tingle. Oh, boy. I have horrible, terrifying associations with tingling.

I have to pee.

I hate to interrupt the process to go to the bathroom.

I might miss something.

But I can't focus on anything else except my bladder.

Can I consider being relaxed enough to just let it come? That would *really* be living in the present.

But how embarrassing. I can't just release control that way.

Who said we have to stay in control? It's okay to relax control in the appropriate place.

Wait a minute! This *is* the appropriate place, if ever there was one.

What will I wear after?

Little girls don't worry about the future.

God, can I just let it go?

The right clothes will be there. Let it go.

It might even be fun to wear something different.

So, let it go.

I relax and pee. I did it!

And again and every so often--again.

I am proud of it!

I love that I let go of control!

I practically prance up and down in my excitement, sharing my great achievement with the group. What a metaphor for letting go. Here in this room is one of the few places where I'm understood and even congratulated. In the feedback, one man says, "You're an inspiration. You're a woman letting go--delightfully and elegantly."

Bev congratulates me and then directs me to a sponge and a bucket of soapy water.

> *"We learn best by losing ourselves. If we can be strong enough to just forget about who we are for a moment instead of taking ourselves so damn seriously, if we forget about what we think, what we believe, what we want--take the risk of forgetting ourselves--we learn with the grace of a blossoming flower."*
>
> *Read and Rusk,* ***I Want to Change, But I Don't Know How***

CHAPTER THIRTY-ONE

THE DAY AFTER the Cross Over Seminar, Karl and I drove back to Portland talking earnestly about what we wanted. I explained that I no longer felt able to have the sex without some kind of emotional connection. I was also no longer interested in playing the mind games. We agreed to be friends, to date other people. To be lovers on dates if we wanted to. To wish the best for the other ... meaning that we would share and care for the other person's finding "the one."

As we talked, I realized that I could no longer simply slip and slide my way vaguely through conversations with Karl. I was learning how to communicate clearly and concisely, difficult and impossible as it seemed. He pointed out cracks and paradoxes in my statements, and from that I learned how confusedly I expressed my feelings. But I welcomed it, telling myself, *This is all practice and so valuable.*

How often with Jack I had felt that the problem was in his not being able to understand me and my feelings. No bloody wonder he couldn't. I was hopelessly scattered and long-winded in expressing myself--or I was so brief and vague and evasive that he couldn't possibly have formed a clear picture of what was going on for me.

So now, with Karl, I worked through my expression--clarifying, becoming more honest, edging closer to my heart connection, all the while realizing, *I cannot overlook the beauty of this difficult gift.*

Alone, after Karl dropped me at home, I thought, *Now what?* Throughout the summer I had continually said to myself, *I want to be alone, to be with God, to read my spiritual books and meditate.* I'd berated myself for being distracted from that focus by spending time in the seminars and relating to Karl--both intellectually and sexually. *Yet,* I realized, *what greater gift of learning could the universe have sent me than the opportunity to learn and grow and to practice how I go about expressing God's essence to my fellow man?*

As one friend had recently said, "Evidently, relating to people, men in particular, is your path." And Jan Paul had said, "Do you have to compartmentalize the different aspects of your life? Couldn't you be spiritual when you are doing these other things?"

The irony, of course, was that it was because I wanted to relate spiritually to people that I sought to spend time in spiritual contemplation and study. *The balances must be possible. The time for that inward looking has been there before, and it can/will be there again.*

As I perambulated my neighborhood loop that night, muscle spasms and old fears surged. I knew that pushing and not taking time--for God, and for peacefulness--was catching up with me. Although I was saddened to lose Karl's lovemaking, I truly felt ready to move on to WHATEVER, or whoever, was next. *After all,* I told myself, *You've been saying, "I want time to read and to meditate." So now you will have it ...*

Oh, my. Every time I invited quiet, inward turning, my imaginings were unprepared for the acute ways that it would manifest. The pendulum would soon swing me far from the summer seminars and delights of Karl into the deepest isolation I had yet experienced. Incorporating the changes set in motion during that summer would require struggle and commitment. The stripping-away process that began in Cross Over was about to assault the deepest layers of my being. Beliefs and expectations would be turned upside-down and I would never view myself or the world the same again.

> *"Think of me therefore at all times: remember thou me and fight. And with mind and reason on me, thou shalt in truth come to me."*
>
> **Bhagavad Gita**, *8;7*

PART V

THERE IS NO TOMORROW

There is no tomorrow. It's only what you have right now.

Peter Dane, ex-lover

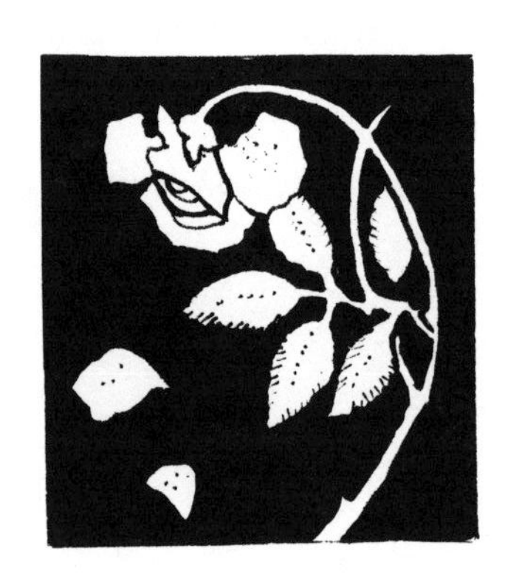

CHAPTER THIRTY-TWO

ASPIRES, THE THIRD level of the seminar trainings, met at six o'clock Tuesday mornings. The gatherings provided on-going reinforcement of the processes and changes begun in the PES and Cross Over. I used Aspires as a practice ground where I could continue evolving and developing those new behaviors which would better serve me.

At the first Aspires meeting I attended, we focused on attachment. How appropriate! Since leaving Cross Over two weeks before, I'd had some sad moments whenever I thought about the lost closeness with Karl. Paradoxically, I was also at peace with letting him go, with releasing the attachment. The sadness was not so much for losing Karl, but for losing "the hunk," and the attention. *But there is so much more ahead where I'm going*, I told myself.

I kept reminding myself that Karl was Wichita, Kansas, and I was going to New York--as per Jan Paul's metaphor of Karl being a station stop along my way to bigger and better things. The image delightfully fit my awareness of my present state, that of opening up my options in the direction of other men.

A lunch visit with Peter, whom I'd not seen for several months, helped affirm for me the extent to which I had blossomed in new directions. Our meeting took place in a cozy restaurant and was a meaningful, close connection. It was also one of the few times that Peter spoke directly to me about our puzzling relationship. As we ate our meal, we shared what was going on for each of us--I with my old story of the health and my body's messages. How I kept looking at this group and that organization and that retreat and this lecture to be signposts and signals and tools for me. How I continued to race about, my body taking me just so far, seemingly healing, and then I'd have a backsliding, discouraging phase.

"It's not external," said Peter. "The message is the same as it was five years ago. Trust yourself. What's inside. The body reminds you to be here now."

He continued, "You're always looking for what's 'out there'--or 'tomorrow.' There is no tomorrow. It's only what you have right now. You get attached to the goals. It's good to want the healing, to want to grow, to want to change. But the *attachment* to the wanting gets in the way."

"How do I stop being this way?"

"Here is a task. Check in with what you're getting. Ask 'Am I getting what I want?' Do this throughout the day. Rather than focusing on the negatives and on what you're *not* getting, form the habit of noticing when you *are* getting what you want--and what it is."

"What I want is wholeness," I said, "to be healthy on all levels--mentally, physically, emotionally, spiritually."

"It can't come from outside."

"But I want help! Teachers, groups, workshops, experts, some guidance to give me the tools for achieving those things." Even as I spoke, I was thinking, *The truth is that I **do** have it within me. It's all about trusting myself--just as all the books and teachers and seminars say.*

As we walked to our cars, Peter said, "I wasn't happy with the way I was with you the last time we were together." He was referring to when he'd come over and out of the blue said, "I want to make love to you." I'd been bowled over because we had scrupulously kept sex out of the interaction since the close time of three years before. I'd also, by then, released most of my emotions toward him. My answer had been, "I'm tired. I'm not sure that I want reinvolvement on this level. Perhaps another time."

Now he said, "I was coming from a needy place. I'd gotten into confused messages toward you. I feel that I was out of integrity. But I thought that you handled it well, that you were coming from an integrous place."

That was probably the most direct acknowledgement he'd ever given me. I smiled and honestly replied, "It was a gift. Because you gave me the opportunity to really act from my core and to be clear about my motives and what I wanted."

The next morning at Aspires I asked for someone to help me bathe the cats and lo! I got an offer--and from Richard Howard, who unbeknown to me was a veterinarian! He came over the next afternoon and the lucky cats received the most thorough and professional bath of their lives. What an example of "asking for what you want," and getting so much more. The cats, I fear, did not appreciate it.

At the next week's Aspires meeting, we did a process in which we shared "Why I am hiding out." For me it was because of fear of imposition--which, I guess, implied fear of rejection. More often than not, I chose not to speak out at Aspires. In PES I had shared a lot, but since Cross Over I had hesitated. I feared I'd express myself awkwardly, with too much explanation, that I wouldn't say it clearly or "right," that no one would be interested ...

As I examined this, the truth dawned. I was awkward and isolated on Tuesday mornings because I was stepping into foreign territory--that of learning a new way to express myself. I was leaving behind old habits of thinking and planning ahead how or what I would say. I was learning how to get away from my head and to talk out of my self-trusting center. *No wonder I've felt clumsy and rough*! I exclaimed. *It's all unfamiliar. I've not done that before--very often.*

And, if I were honest, I could see that I truly was developing a higher level of self-trust. More and more often I was able to be calm and present while others were talking. When my turn came I spoke with relatively little head-preparation. Awkwardly for sure, and I wanted to express myself better. But I could tell that I'd already improved. There was more calm, less shakiness throughout my body, slower speech, clearer communication.

> *"We do not go straight up the side of the mountain on this trip. We circle it, slowly, carefully, sometimes losing our footing, sometimes back-tracking because we've reached an impasse. Many times we have stumbled, but as we grow in understanding, as we rely more and more on our inner strength, available for the taking, we become more sure-footed."*
>
> *from,* ***Each Day a New Beginning***

CHAPTER THIRTY-THREE

HOPING TO GAIN some sort of insight into my direction and purpose, I scheduled, and eagerly anticipated, an appointment with a well-known psychic. The result of the meeting turned out nothing like my expectations and was, in fact, the beginning of another process.

When I entered his office, the psychic, a young man, was sitting like an executive with his feet on his large desk. Introducing myself, I said, "The reason I'm here is because I'm interested in more clarity about my work, my relationships, my health, about where I'm headed."

He unfolded his long narrow frame from the chair and said, "You don't need to be here. Everything is fine with you. Just trust yourself, your heart. What you're doing is fine. Trust it."

Blank. No clues, hints, directions, no pieces of the puzzle coming together from this guy.

"Let it flow. You're following each thing one step at a time."

"Yeah, that's what everyone says, but I'm so unsure of myself." I grovelled, "Can you at least tell me something about my health?"

"All the clamorings are coming from your head. Listen to your heart. Your health may not be as good as you want it right now, but it's not that bad."

With that he ejected the tape and sent me home, saving me $60, and both of us an evening.

At home I sat in the darkening living room glad of the time to be quiet and without demands. I felt tired and vacant after my aborted appointment. It suddenly occurred to me that maybe the psychic chose not to talk to me because he foresaw some disaster. Perhaps he saw death or an accident. Rather than fill me with negatives, he chose to say nothing.

In the days that followed, I pondered these possibilities. At the end of the week, another incident occurred which provoked still more bouts of questions, doubts, and fears.

Regina, a lady who could read auras, offered to read mine one afternoon. After she had finished, I left the session breathless and distraught. Numbly, I parked the car on a side street. It was impossible to return to work. So this was how it felt to be told, "You are near to being complete in this life," to be told, "There are holes--dry wells in your aura, as if someone's sucked it dry."

The information was powerful, staggering, yet not surprising. Regina had seen: "Anger. Pain. Black smudges in the aura." She told me, "You're searching for ways to do it differently, mentally, physically, spiritually. ... You *do* give out unconditional love ... you don't let love in."

That surprised me, because I felt as if I were looking for love all the time, that I was taking, taking and never giving back.

"You get impatient and say 'I'll do it all myself.' *Ask* for support. *Ask* for love. Why not use the Tuesday mornings at Aspires to learn how? Let go of not asking."

Seeing my expression of consternation, she offered, "I'll stand up with you if you like."

Then, looking directly into my eyes, Regina said, "Leaving this planet is a choice. You can decide that you're complete and that you want to go on to other places. Or even if you get complete, you could choose to stay around for a while."

Stay around for a while? Leave the planet?

Suddenly viewing my time as precious and limited, I grew clearer, sharper, more concise. I wanted to drop all the abstractions in my life. All the things that I was doing which were not clean, or which were tinged with distaste, doubt, or without integrity. *Can I stop concerning myself with non-essentials, trivialities, vanity?*

Back at the Whole Health Center, dazedly lying face down on the exam table, I processed this new way of viewing my life. Worries about my budget, about paying my bills, about my muscle tone, dissipated. I opened to trust. *I **can** let go of the old ways, the* *postponing of my healing, the hiding out, the protection,* I told myself. *Let people see me, who I am, that I am hurting, that I'm in pain, and feel isolated in it. The lesson is now, not tomorrow.*

> *"It is almost as though we were never completely born, so much of ourselves is suppressed and compacted just beneath the surface. So much of ourselves postponed ... To become wholly born, whole beings, we must stop postponing life. To the degree we postpone life, we postpone death."*
>
> *Stephen Levine,* ***Who Dies?***

Since Cross Over, I had been seeing Steve Hillinger, the firewalk leader, on a counseling basis. Despite the $50 per session outlay, I felt that I had to pursue my commitment to self-growth. I saw learning to sleep as a big part of that, and after three sessions with Steve, the sleep was doing much better.

The afternoon after my aura reading, I related to Steve the psychic and Regina's words, and that I had started using the terminology "If I have 60 days to live." Steve quietly listened and guided me, again, to myself.

"Do you *want* to live beyond 60 days?"

After a long silence, I answered, "I *think* so."

Why is it not definite? I wondered. I had no images of beyond 60 days, of my birthday or of Christmas, no image of purpose, of people, men, lovers, or of career or work that I wanted to do. *My only purpose right now is to connect with my whole, my spiritual self. Everything outside of that seems extraneous and unappealing.*

Scrunching my eyes closed to hold back the tears, I murmured, "Even if I died, what difference would it make? It would be nice to at least have people miss me when I die."

"Stand up more and share."

"That's exactly what Regina said! To share with the Tuesday morning people what's really going on for me."

"Sharing who you are with the people in Aspires will be a release. Keeping in the pain is a way of holding on to it."

I mumbled, "My experience has been that talking about my health and my pain is an imposition. People don't want to hear it. There is no way they can empathize. The illness separates and isolates and disconnects me."

"You'll be surprised. That's been your experience and it's possible that there is another experience."

"I'm sure people hearing me talk about my body think, 'She's a hypochondriac. She's fishing for love and attention.'"

"I absolutely know that all those people in Aspires are just champing at the bit to empathize with you. I would bet all I own that you'll be surprised."

"Every time I think about standing before the Aspires people and sharing my pain and fear, the tension runs down my body. It is too blatant. Standing in front of them and expressing my grief and pain is like *asking* to be cradled."[1]

"What's wrong with that?"

I had no answer except that it was terribly fearful to lay myself on the line showing a need, asking outright for cradling.

Taking my hand, Steve gently asked, "Do you know the gifts you give?"

"No."

"What I get from you is a mirror. I get to remind myself as I remind you. You give me the gift of your courage. I get the gift of your passion to find your spiritual self."

Two days later I got a bit of a shock. In the morning a skin cancer on my nose was removed with laser surgery. The procedure was painless, but I was unprepared for the indented spot on the side of my nose. I was also surprised when the nurse put a large white bandage across my nose and instructed, "Leave it on until tomorrow night."

I had to laugh at the situation. The next morning was to be my Big Unveiling at Aspires ... the momentous day when Barbara Marie stepped out of hiding and revealed her solemnest self--with a bright white beak.

That evening, walking in the cool autumn haze, I was full of nervousness about the morrow and questioned what I would say. *Ah! That's the lesson,* I realized. *I'll say exactly what is perfect for me in the moment.* ***How*** *it is perceived is not the goal. The point is for* ***me*** *to have the experience of sharing that part of me. So that others--and I--will experience the* ***real*** *me, a person who can be who*

---

1 Process of lying back in the arms of several people and being "cradled" while music plays.

I am without fearing rejection, disapproval and isolation.

> *"One must learn*
> *By doing the thing: for though you*
> *think you know it*
> *You have no certainty, until you try."*
> *Sophocles,* ***Trachiniae***

That night I slept hardly at all, full of the awareness of my morning revelation. I arrived at Aspires very nervous, very inward and somber, in dull contrast to the happy room, full of balloons and greetings, for Gene who was retiring.

Steve and Regina sat near me occasionally holding my hand or grasping my shoulder in gestures of support. Finally my turn came. Regina stood up with me, embracing me from behind. I gave my talk, legs shaking, blinking back tears. The group of people before me seemed to merge into one mass. I had no sense of them as individuals.

When I'd finished, the facilitator approached me and asked, "What does their support look like to you?"

I was quaking with nervousness and all I could think of saying was, "I guess if people would ask me how I am."

He said, "If you give them the message that you want privacy, they'll respect that."

When the group broke up, I felt adrift. What would I do now? I managed to connect with a few people. Some approached me. Not many. Lewis. Jan. Steve. I told Steve, "I didn't do it right. I didn't say what I wanted."

He hugged me and said, "You did it perfectly. I was listening."

I was grateful for his support. How I longed to be so full of integrity, so acting out of my core as he was. How could I then guess that one day I would be able to support Steve? Tomorrow's strengths are forged from today's trials. They are always with us, only waiting to be recognized and drawn forth.

CHAPTER THIRTY-FOUR

THREE DAYS HAD passed since my last session with Steve Hillinger, and I was feeling utterly depressed. The day had been like a marathon of playing musical doctors. I'd started out already discouraged after a sleepless night, and throughout the long waits and the doctors' offices and the examinations, I kept wondering, *What can be the point in a life which goes on and on in this kind of pain?* As I crisscrossed the city in ever descending depths of discouragement I kept remembering, ***I do** have choice.*

In the morning, Nancy, the massage therapist who could see visions, took one look at me on the table and said, "This body doesn't care whether it lives or dies." Later, at Dr. Singh's, I felt hollow and frustrated at the obstacles that showed up in my exam. Then Dr. Parker, the cranial specialist, found numerous problems with my jaw that could affect my spinal nerves. Paula, the nutritionist, read my computer print-out, and said, "You're out of my league."

Back at Dr. Singh's to discuss Paula's report, I was quivering with emotion. He reassured me, "Everything is reversible."

Part of me believed it and another part felt only despair, because I'd slogged through months of pills and bills and strict diets, and I still had subnormal health.

After leaving Dr. Singh's, without an eyeblink, I stepped into a phone booth and rang the airline to cancel the next month's Mexico trip. I'd tried so hard to believe it could happen, but I couldn't pretend any more. No matter how much I desired to be normal or tried to be positive, I couldn't fabricate the health or the gusto for the journey.

How the tables turn. On that dismal day as I canceled my dream of the Mexico holiday, I had no inkling that I was in fact opening a space for its eventual fruition--in joy and companionship far surpassing my then limited desires and imaginings.

Do I want to spend my last 60 days traipsing from doctor to doctor? That's what I wondered as I ploughed through a day such as that one. *I could be at Breitenbush right now, learning to love myself and be calm. Instead, am I spinning my wheels on yet another form of external distraction?*

Like a litany, I kept remembering, *I have choice. I'll give it two months. THEN I'll CHOOSE.*

Questions and speculations and daily notations about my body were my constant companions. *Is that too self-focused?* I wondered. *Or is it necessary in order to clearly explain what's going on?* I was thoroughly tired of restricted diets. I speculated that I'd be more motivated if I could see them making some difference. These were my thoughts as I walked, and they were followed by the pleasant thought, *I have choice. I can choose this or not.* It was a sweet realization.

As I pursued the process of living as if I only had 60 days, my priorities got very clear. If I had limited time I bloody well didn't want to spend it making bridal bouquets--or losing weight, or worrying about how big or small my body was. I decided that I might as well relish the food that came to me in this period, without guilt, fear or reservation.

How I looked no longer mattered as it once had. Spending time preoccupied with face and vanity seemed silly. I chose not to return for a better permanent even though it would have been free. *Why did I spend two and a half hours of my life changing my hair???*

The new wicker furniture in my living room didn't delight me as it once had long ago in my imagination. Did it really matter what kind of curtains I hung or whether I hung any at all? On the other hand, I figured that I might as well enjoy living in beautiful surroundings and seeing the place looking as nice as I'd always dreamed. *Is that being selfish?*

If I had 60 days to live I certainly wouldn't spend them working at the Whole Health Center. Instead, I would go to Breitenbush Hot

Springs for two weeks, or to the Healing and Learning Center in Eugene. I would concentrate on healing, and on finding some sort of spiritual awareness.

It was obvious what I must do. I decided that when Victor returned from his latest trip to England I would tell him I wanted to withdraw. *There is something more for me and I'm not getting it now. I don't have time to patiently try one process and then another sandwiched between working hours or on weekends. The issue is NOW!*

> *"As for the right time to act? The time, inevitably, is now. It can only be now. Truth has no special time of its own."*
>
> *Albert Schweitzer, from* ***Albert Schweitzer's Mission*** *by Norman Cousins.*

Living as if I only had 60 days became the main thread of my existence. I wrote reams, read, meditated. More than ever before, I was cutting through the obsolete beliefs about how I "should" live and opening up to living how I *wanted* to. Peter's statement that there is no tomorrow was my theme, and I lived it in each moment of each day. There were times when I felt utterly alone, when I longed for some sort of guidance. But how could I ask for help, for what I needed, when I myself didn't know how anyone else could give it to me? I thought on the privacy of pain, how no one can possibly share that experience with another person.

What is the point? I kept asking myself. *Why am I here to spend my time withdrawing ever more from people, events, the world?* My body seemed to be deteriorating before my eyes. I felt suffocatingly trapped in it and utterly helpless to stop the disintegration. My thoughts were preoccupied with death. Each time I monitored my legs, noticed the stiffness, felt the unrelenting "crab" in my back, each time I looked at my increasingly flabby body, I thought, *How shall I end it?* And I'd wonder, *Whatever happened to joy in living? To happiness? To whom can I turn except myself?* To reveal my despair to others seemed a pointless imposition.

My mind said, *There's life to be led! I want to be out and about! I want to be on with it! To counsel, to teach, to share. I want to be with people and laugh and dance and have a job that supports me and fills me with purpose.* I wanted to go about my day feeling like singing and not hesitating to take on tasks like bookkeeping, dish washing or bathing the cats. But the body said, *Rest. The energy is not here. The alacrity is dull.* All I could do was honor the body's messages and try to be thankful for the quiet time to retreat, rest and regroup.

I berated myself for being a miserable failure at trusting, at turning negatives into positives. My self-confidence sputtered to non-existence. I felt incapable of making decisions on my own. Talking to others, however, was just as confusing. Everybody wanted to be helpful, so they promoted *their* chiropractor, herbalist, M.D., or seminar ...

> *"You may feel overwhelmed with exhaustion from meeting obstruction upon obstruction in your passage. Yet you always have a choice, you can see all this apparent negativity as "bad luck" or you can recognize it as an obstacle course, a challenge peculiar to the initiation you are presently undergoing. Then each setback, each humiliation becomes a test of character. When your inner being is shifting and reforming on a deep level, patience, constancy and perseverance are called for. So stay centered, see the humor, and keep on keeping on."*
>
> *The Rune of Initiation, from* ***The Book of Runes***

Then dawned a day when I felt certain that something was at last shifting. For the first time, I attended the much talked about Sunday morning "Celebration" at the Living Enrichment Center. By evening I was full of buoyant energy.

When I had arrived that morning, the school gym where the gathering was held was bursting with a vivacious crowd of people noisily milling and hugging and greeting each other. There was some singing and then the leader, Mary Boggs, began to speak. She talked about the need for a "flood" in our lives, something to clean us out and help us leave the old behind so that we can move forward cleansed and reborn into the realm of inner trust and wholeness, into that place where we all are longing to be. Sometimes it takes a flood to get us there.

Her words moved me, as did her clear and vivid presentation, so human, so heartful. She said, "We all want to move on, but because of fear of what will happen, we may not, until we let loose of the rope that holds us in place."

When Mary finished speaking, I felt at once purged and full, her words had touched me so profoundly. The hour closed with a young man at the piano singing a song titled *I Want To Live*. Then the tears streamed. The words echoed my innermost urge--with which I'd nearly lost touch. It was as if the entire service had been directed at me.

"I want to live
I want to grow
I want to see
I want to know
I want to share what I can give
I want to live."
John Denver

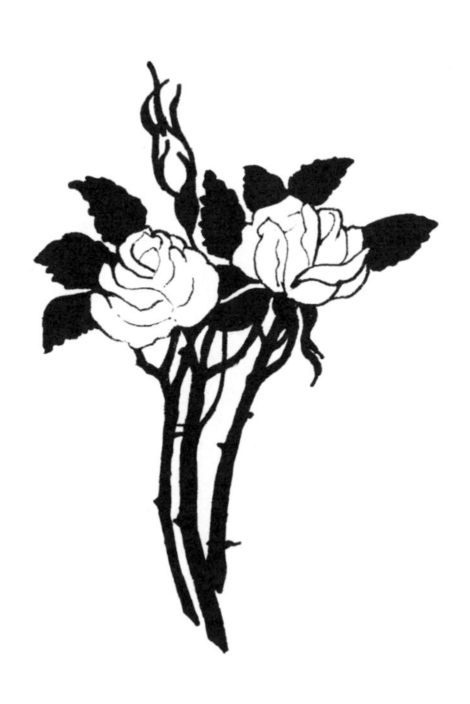

CHAPTER THIRTY-FIVE

SEVERAL DAYS HAD passed since the "Celebration" at the Living Enrichment Center, and an occasion occurred which reflected the new lightness that was beginning to flicker within me. I attended the opera with John Honse, the gentle and witty cherub from my PES. I couldn't have guessed, when I asked John to join me, that he'd once been considered for managing the San Francisco Opera, or that he wrote oratorios in his spare time. The music had been exuberant and rousing. The melodies lyrical and haunting. The performers and the production impeccable! I came away feeling enlivened, alive!

And John was delightful, heart-filled, sweet, open, honest. He gave such acknowledgement as I'd not had since Jan Paul.

He appreciated my blue outfit--the skirt and silk blouse picked out by Jan Paul. The silver jewelry. My hair. At dinner, John said, "You look like a certain Egyptian goddess."

And, "Your power is like water."

"How is water powerful?"

"Without mentioning the Grand Canyon ... It's the ability to be held in any shape or situation or to mold to the situation to fit with it. Like water, you're able to fit to the situation ... to give back to the people you're with what it is that they need at that moment."

"The Chinese say that water is the most powerful element, because it is perfectly nonresistant ..."

Florence Scovel Shinn, from ***Each Day a New Beginning***

At my next visit with Steve, another shift occurred. I was lamenting my situation, saying, "I am frustrated and feel such a lack because I *want* to work. I want to be inspired and motivated as I perceive you and others are. But my body lets me do so much and then I crash. It's exasperating to have to rest all the time."

Steve had said, "You know, you're one of the lucky ones."

At first it was hard to see it that way, but then the idea grew, and I began to see my situation differently.

So many people were locked into *having* to toil, *having* to support themselves. Here was I not *having* to do either one. What I was "choosing" (ha-ha) was to heal. But by "choosing" not working, I found myself adrift, out of sync with the world's ways. Not knowing how, where, or what my calling was, I felt a void in my life.

Later, sitting alone with Betty in the living room, I began allowing myself to rejoice in my stay-home situation. *Acceptance! To relax and revel in the freedom and the time to grow and simply let it happen.* I told myself, *I release yearning to be off working and purposeful like the people I admire.* ***This*** *is my purpose now. Other purposes will reveal themselves when the time is right.*

And they have, and do. How could I imagine the far-flung and stimulating directions in which my purpose would one day lead me, or how joyfully I would embrace it? All, of course, completely removed from my own tradition and the usual ways of working. With each year, I shed more layers of expectations and beliefs about how I should work, serve, be in the world.

> *"And do thy duty, even if it be humble, rather than another's even if it be great. To die in one's duty is life: to live in another's is death."*
>
> **Bhagavad Gita**, *3:35*

A week later I was chatting on the phone with a friend, when all at once excitement welled within me. I was saying, "What I really want to do is counseling, but you must have credentials--" Suddenly I stopped, realizing that I *could* get credentials, that I *could* do the necessary schooling, that I *could* afford to stop working. I'd not even thought about it, I had been so oppressively stuck in the idea that I *had* to work.

If I severed my ties with the Whole Health Center once and for all, I would be able to devote all my time to healing and to learning through experiential trainings like Cross Over and PES back-up teams, Neurolinguistic Programming trainings, massage courses, counseling, etc. Maybe I would someday lead seminars or counsel `a la Jan Paul or the Wings trainers, or Steve Hillinger ... maybe even lead firewalks! I felt as if the clouds had instantly swept away from in front of the sun.

And a week later, the first sign of my new course materialized. A friend phoned and asked me if I would be willing to see her friend who was battling candida. You bet!

The big day of my first counselling session with my first candida client came. I was keenly aware that this was perhaps the beginning of a new career. The session flew past and extended to another hour. After the woman left, I broke into songs and danced around the house hugging myself and beaming. I *knew* I had given her valuable information and options and that I had supported her. Before the woman left, she made another appointment and her comment was, "It's so good to find someone who understands!" My confidence level soared and satisfaction infused every pore of my being.

A week before Halloween I did something different and drove out to Sauvie Island. I wanted to break the pattern of my days by taking time away from the battleground of interior struggles and skirmishes. Goldens, reds, rusts, browns; these were the colors of the autumn island. Such a gift it was--to thread through the crackling rows of golden corn stalks silhouetted against a domed azure sky. At the beach I was perfectly, peacefully alone. The air was clear enough to see the white peaked mountains--St. Helens' flattened dome, Mt. Adams, Mt. Hood--beyond the calm river. Sitting on the sand in the sun, I meditated, soothed by the lapping of the waves that sprang up each time a boat passed.

On my way home I discovered the Pumpkin Patch. How could I have waited ten years to do so? It was an autumn institution with its fields of vivid orange pumpkins and the throngs of child-filled cars rolling in and out. I threw myself into the moment, getting carried away buying bundles of colorful squashes to take home and pile in baskets on my front porch. My car was laden with gold and green striped Delicatas, mottled exotic turbans, Hubbards in brilliant oranges, dark greens, sherbets, and yes, a pumpkin.

At home that night I sat cozily by the fire feeling at once mellow and energetic. My journal was, as always, within reach. Betty busily did her booper things about the room. I picked up my pen and started writing. In two minutes this poem popped out:

TO BETTY BOOP

Betty comes booping
Trundling and swooping
Little wee beastie
Out on a lark.

A furry cadenza
Flies fondly and freely
On to my lap
And into my heart.

I was glad the next afternoon that I went to see Steve. I had planned to let this be my last session but, as we got into it, I knew that the time with him was too valuable. I hadn't known what I'd talk about. But out it flowed, my picture of life.

"It's not easy for me to let it be simple. My vision of life is struggle. Life is walking along under cliffs with teetering boulders and the Road Runner is up there waiting to push them over."

"What's happening when it's simple?"

"I get anxious, uncomfortable. I expect something's going to happen next. I heal a little bit and then fear, what's the Road Runner got in store for me next?"

"How do you know when it's simple?"

"Because it's *too* easy. I feel uncomfortable, as if something's bound to go wrong if I'm not struggling or working at it."

Steve smiled, "I don't think you're ready to give that one up. Why do you cling to it?"

"It's been the way I've identified myself for the last fifteen years--twenty years--maybe most of my life. You know, `Life's a bitch and then you die.'"

"I want to be sure you want to give it up because you want to, not because you should or you know it would be good for you or you have to. Play with it for the week. The operative word is *play*."

How knowing Steve was. He knew that my tendency would be to

dwell on such issues as on a sore tooth, and I really wanted to drop that old belief. It was a very deeply rooted one. Once it was vanquished my life would be simple, totally different. Could I face that? *The thought of a simple, struggle-free life scares me!* I realized. *How can that be? Then there'd be no loopholes, no reasons for not being terrific! No excuses for not living up to my potential. And I'd lose my identity--I wouldn't know who I am.*

> *"Struggle however, is not natural; it is an unholy battle we fight with ourselves."*
>
> *Stuart Wilde,* ***Life Was Never Meant to be a Struggle***

The following day I was invited to join a group at a mediation evening at a counselor's house. When it was over, I drove home grinning and singing and chuckling in amazement at how incredibly the evening had synchronized with Steve's session of the day before. The woman counselor had guided us in a meditation in which we walked to cabinets along hallways. The cabinets contained old memories and tapes ... many items that we wanted to clear out. We could see ourselves roller-skating down a clear, open corridor.

I had the image that I'd discussed with Steve, of the Road Runner up on the cliff waiting with a plank to push down the teetering boulder. Suddenly I just blew it up--"phewff!" Brown and buff pieces of rock, plank, and Road Runner all exploded in a paisley pattern against the sky. That myth was gone!

When things are going well, I told myself, *I will no longer look for the boulder that is waiting to fall on me. Instead, I will have the image of the rocks flying through the air and I'll hear the "phewff!" of them exploding.* I even had a 3" X 5" yellow card with them symbolized on it ... my gift of insight drawn by the man who had been my partner that evening.

Surely this was one of the major issues that had been waiting to be resolved on my field of battle. I couldn't possibly proceed to become and do all that I wanted if I continually created obstacles to my progress.

> *"Sometimes it takes great effort to discover that life was meant to be effortless."*
>
> *Rusty Berkus,* ***Appearances***

A week later, talking with Trish while she massaged me, I knew that I needed to let the child part of me out. I was much too serious about all this healing and personal growth stuff. I commented to Trish, "You know, if it seems like work, then it can't be what I'm looking for anyway."

Trish nodded in agreement and then asked, "What do you expect to gain from reading all those books?"

"Understanding."

She shook her head, "The understanding you want isn't in the books. Take a vacation. Have fun for two weeks."

Leaving Trish, I drove to the nearby deli to meet Jack. I decided to pretend that I was on vacation and that I didn't have to eat at home. I splurged on a real bread sandwich and a bottle of vegy juice. How delightfully frivolous and tasty.

From the deli Jack took me to see his new house--so perfect for him, with lots of character and possibilities. It sat against a backdrop of Iron Mountain rock formations which afforded excellent opportunities for him to implement exciting landscape designs.

As I prepared to leave, I told Jack, "I'm pretending I'm on vacation. I'm going to indulge in an early movie. Would you like to join me?"

He said, "That sounds good, but why not rent a couple of videos?"

I'd never done such a thing. In fact, I'd been wondering why, and what, were all those stores sprouting up with Video signs on them. Off we went.

In the video shop, "Jack, I'm bowled over. It's like a giant library of movies."

"See how nice it is?"

"I could watch all the movies that I've missed. How much does a VCR cost?"

With Jack's enthusiastic encouragement, we first picked out two movies, and then scooted off to the appliance store. Jack happily guided me in choosing what I needed, a VCR *and* a color T.V., since my old one was black and white. *Might as well go whole hog. After all, I'm on vacation.* Within two hours we were back at the house moving my furniture about in readiness for the big installation.

The last week in October I embarked on a course which would have far-reaching influences on my life. I began attending the weekly meditation class that Steve went to. It was held in the office of Mike Gotesman, a MSW (Master Social Worker) in Beaverton. I came home from the first evening with more recognitions of the rightness of the path I was on. Mike was another one of those powerful people who was successful and purposeful, but who let his life be run by tuning into something other/bigger within himself. Talking and meditating with Mike and the group seemed right, as if I had come home.

I didn't know it, but I'd found the support I'd longed for--in the form of Mike and the other seven class members. Not only did we cultivate the art of meditation but with ruthless insight, gentleness, humor and honesty, Mike nudged each one of us into breaking through our barriers and beliefs into ever deeper areas of inner trust.

In hindsight, I can see that with the embarkation on my association with Mike and the class there was an imperceptible upswing on every level of my life. Although I wouldn't realize it for some time, there was no longer any question of what I would choose in 60 days. In retrospect, I can bless that period of living as if I only had limited time. It was a valuable process at age 40 for examining and cutting through the peripheral clutter which obscured my true priorities. How many of us postpone such self-awareness until we're in our eighties--or until it's too late?

"But to be forgetful of death is to be forgetful of life, whereas thinking of one's death is an act in which life begins once more to appear as a source of light. A man who knows death also knows life. The converse is true; the man who is forgetful of death, is forgetful of life also."

*Ladislaus Boros, in **The Scent of Roses** by Mary O'Hara*

CHAPTER THIRTY-SIX

THROUGHOUT THE WINTER the seed was germinating. Gigantic growth was underway, but it was outwardly invisible. Like a child running daily to check a box of seedlings, I checked the usual places to measure my growth--health, body, relationships, abundance, career, sense of spiritual connection--and was perpetually dissatisfied. I know now that transmutation *was* taking place but, like the seed, it was hidden, and thus not very satisfying to the ego, or, I fear, to readers.

Hours and days rolled by in silent contemplation: walking, cooking, attending classes, reading, studying. Every circumstance became grist for my healing mill. I wrote reams as I continually opened myself to some Something within and sought to incorporate it into my everyday life.

The chronicle of those inner workings and insights is available in another accounting. Here, I have chosen to share only the more visible (and more readable) experiences of this germination process.

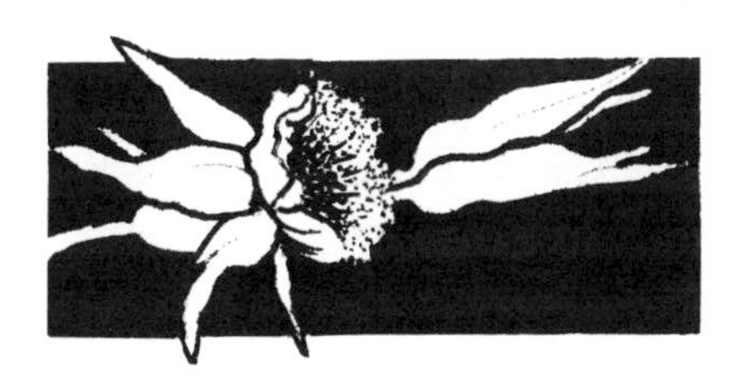

It was the first week of November. Since I'd been too tired to go to the Wing's Halloween Party, I decided to dress up for Aspires on Tuesday morning. I'd so looked forward to sharing my costume, and I didn't want to wait another year to do so. I wore my "I SKIED MT. ST. HELENS" T shirt--which was peppered with burned out holes--my knickers, burnt sox and tennies, and dark blue beret covered with "ash" (buckwheat flour). Buoyantly, I drove to Aspires singing *I've Got To Be Me.* People responded well, laughing and grinning and hugging me.

After the meeting, joining the others for breakfast at the restaurant--in my outfit--I felt high and happy and grateful, and aware that I'd accessed *some* well-being state. No thought about how I was coming across, whether I was foolish or saying the wrong thing. Just there. Being. I had so much fun that I wore the costume up to the university for my hypnosis session with Dr. Hale.

"The point is to learn to season life's banquet with those redolent spices of stress and risk."

Read and Rusk, ***I Want to Change, But I Don't Know How***

Early the next morning, I stood a long time gazing out of my bedroom window. Below me, the garage roof, the garden, and the undisturbed neighborhood gleamed transformed under soft white blankets. There were no sounds of the morning. The sky, too, shimmered softly with greys and peaches backdropping the silhouettes of the tall dark trees. When the snow arrives, I'm always filled with wonderment and delight. Gathering up the cats, I threw them outside and watched, chuckling, as they tentatively explored this unfamiliar and magic world.

My energy was up so, despite the snow, I negotiated the encrusted roads and drove to the pool. As I splashed down and back along my lap lane, I kept dwelling on Shakespeare's line, "There is nothing either good or bad, but thinking makes it so." I felt drawn to reading Shakespeare. I remembered other lines. "This above all else, to thine own *self* be true ..." I began to think of Shakespeare in a new way, as a spiritually expressive being.

Nothing is good or bad, I repeated, as I cut through the water ... *Butter is not good or bad. Swimming three quarters of a mile is not good or bad. Weighing five pounds more or less is not good or bad.*

Working, money, health, being married or single, young or old --are not good or bad. It's just my ***thinking*** *that perceives these things as being one way or the other.*

A few days later, I attended a sweat lodge ceremony on the Sandy River. I had gone without expectations and came away uplifted, in touch with the same kind of feelings I had had at the firewalk--feelings of release, of letting go of fears and illusions, at least in those moments.

My girl friend, Anne, and I arrived at the site around ten o'clock in the morning. Killing time waiting for the fire to be ready, I walked beside the full, rollicking river and up through the wooded lots. The river was banked by a sturdy clay cliff on the other side with trees marching right up from the cliff top into the sky. I didn't know it, but two years later I would be living there.

With regard to the details of the sweat ceremony, much was left unsaid. I asked as many questions as I could of the leader in an attempt to be informed enough not to glitch it up for myself or others.

"What happens if I need to leave?"

"You're not supposed to. You get permission from Amy, the leader. You overcome your fears--go beyond your comfort zone. Stretch yourself, but if you feel light-headed or dizzy you should leave."

"You can't drink any water while you're in the lodge."

"What if I have to pee?"

"Not likely once you're sweating, but you can ask."

We entered the lodge for four "rounds." One for the west, when we invoked the spirits to come and be with us. One for the north, which was represented by the color black. Here we prayed to release our burdens and to be given certain things. Then east. Then south and sky and earth.

Before entering, we had all been given bits of fabric in white, black, red, green and yellow which represented the earth, and a blue for the sky. They also represented the six directions--north, south, east, west, up, down. We filled the fabric pieces with tobacco and tied them in little bundles with strings and attached a silent prayer or blessing of our choice to each one. Inside the lodge, we each hung our string of prayer pieces up on the roof limbs to be left there.

After each round the lodge door was to be open, we could look out and breath fresh air. At that time, also, new hot stones were conveyed in on bleached deer antlers and added to the stones already in the pit.

The leader issued us each a voluminous sheet in which to wrap ourselves. Then we each ducked through the entry into the lodge, saying as our turn came, "Ho! Ma-ta-ke-asi!" We continued to repeat this whenever a new hot stone was added, when we prayed, when someone made some comment that elicited punctuation, and when it was time to crawl out of the lodge.

In the first round I felt like a roasting marshmallow blistering over a fire. I became uncomfortably hot and had a great deal of trouble breathing. Bending my head down to the earth, I turned around so I could breath the air entering from under the hem of the lodge coverings. That round must have lasted 25 minutes.

In the second round I began to wonder why I would want to come back for the third and fourth rounds. I had nothing I needed to prove and was having a horrific time breathing. My body was smothering in the heat and I felt I couldn't get clean air in my lungs. Mightily relieved when Amy opened the door, I told the group that this was decision time for me, as I was experiencing questions about why should I go through more of this.

We were allowed to go outside and walk around, to drink water, or even dunk in the icy river. The air and the river revived me although, after the river dunking, I experienced a rush of lightheadedness. I thought, *Oh no, now I really have the toxins dashing around. I could definitely do damage once I go back inside.* All these fears in spite of the fact that I was the one in the group who prayed for releasing my preoccupation with the body. Yet there I was suffering and fearing away.

I drank water and stood by the fire outside the lodge. The man who'd been introduced as a veterinarian knelt there getting ready to shovel away more hot rocks. Smiling up at me, he said, "Know that it's perfect if you decide to stop now." He added, "No one has ever died in a sweat lodge."

For some reason that cleared something up for me. I'd not thought of being afraid of dying so I wondered, *Then what am I afraid of?* I feared not getting enough breath. I knew it was fear that was making me so conscious of my discomfort. *Fear of what? Death? But I know I won't die!*

So back in I went. By now the lodge was cooled down and very comfortable. The vet had said, "You'll be cooler sitting directly on the sand," so I removed the carpet fragment that I'd originally been sitting on. That immediately made a difference.

Somebody else had said, "Don't focus on the body. That's what mantras are for. They focus you elsewhere." So I focused on the chanting, on songs that people sang, on my own mantra which was "Nothing is good or bad, but thinking makes it so."

I'd figured out that if I covered my head with my sheet and wrapped it around my nose and mouth it made breathing much easier. It had been that blast of heat on my face and head that was the most uncomfortable. The hot body and the sweat was not bad. I was very calm, felt released totally to letting it be. That round was easy, uplifting, peaceful. I didn't even feel the need for the door to open and, when it did, I was happy to remain seated, calmly breathing in the late afternoon air.

Something had released. Perhaps I got out of my head and into the feeling of knowing that it was only the body, of realizing that it truly was my thinking that perceived it as good or bad, hot or cold, and that thinking aside, there is no effect of heat or cold on the real. Whatever it was, I was peaceful and at ease. The fourth round progressed equally comfortably and it was with a calm sense of joy that I left the lodge and walked naked down to the icy river to rinse away the black sand that caked my body and hair.

Once we were cleaned and dressed, I approached the vet with whom I felt a kinship, and I thanked him for his encouragement. He said, "I've been through so many sweat lodges that I have a sense of other people's discomfort or fear. I can also tell as soon as it shifts. It's often very quick, just like with you."

Gathering in a nearby cabin, we ate the tasty food that everybody had brought. Nice to meet and talk and know these people better. It was eight o'clock before Anne and I threaded our way along the dark dirt road to the car. The stars gleamed sharply bright, the breeze was warm. What a perfect, wondrous day. So unanticipated and so welcome. So much more than I could have dreamed.

"From the world of senses, Arjuna, comes heat and comes cold, and pleasure and pain. They come and they go: they are transient. Arise above them, strong soul."

***Bhagavad Gita**, 2:14*

CHAPTER THIRTY-SEVEN

ON THE MONDAY after the sweat lodge, as I sat quietly, I asked inside, *What should I write to Mom and Dad?*

The answer came, *The sweat lodge.* I remembered the angel card "Sharing" that I had picked out in the last workshop. Sharing myself completely with my parents, holding nothing back, was a big stretch. Mom and Dad had had no clues from me as to the workshops or the study I'd been doing. Now it seemed time to share--regardless of being put down, misunderstood or ignored.

The way for me to affect Mom and Dad's lives is not by my telling them what to do. It's by my example. The only way they can ***know*** *me is if I write or talk about the important issues of my life.* The point of our relationship was not for me to talk about dinners, or dog shows, or the weather. *It's to reveal the deeper side of myself and in so doing they begin to recognize and acknowledge that part of themselves.*

I typed a five page letter about the sweat lodge.

In the middle of my writing, the phone rang. It was Stuart Hall, whom I'd met at the firewalk in June. Now, after six months, out of the blue, he phoned me and poured his heart out. It was about his relationship to Jean, his wife. I felt privileged and honored that he'd thought of me as safe enough to do this with.

I invited him over and at five o'clock he was waiting in the driveway when I returned from a dismal appointment with Dr. Evans. Putting aside my own problems, I spent the next two hours with Stuart. He was totally stuck in despair, anger, resentment and fear. He wanted Jean for his mate, but she didn't want him. *How can I help him?* I kept asking myself. I listened. As often as I could, I remembered to refrain from judging or advising. It was so tempting to want to say, "This is so and this is so, etc." and try to tell him what he must do.

Stuart said, "I called you because I guess I thought what you've been through physically might mean you'd understand."

I knew I gave him a friend to listen to him. That's all I felt I really did. Except to emphasize that he had two choices--gripe or change.

Once Stuart had gone, I remembered Dr. Evans, and I caved in deep down, bereft of support, bewildered. *How do I maintain my sense of positivism when the body is so emphatically calling attention to the negatives?*

I felt clobbered. My thoughts clambered like chattering crows in my head. After all the work I'd done, Dr. Evans told me, "You've got serious auto immune problems." She didn't call it "MS." *What difference does a label make when the body is a wreck?* Had I made wrong decisions as I sought healing? How did I know that seeing Dr. Evans was a "right" decision?

"Diet is important," she had said. "Fats are critical in auto immune disease."

Have I overindulged despite my restraint and feeling deprived all the time?

Dr. Evans also expressed her displeasure in my exploring the TMJ[1] as a possible factor in causing the back pain. She said, "As I adjust you, your system will change. You'll have to change your TMJ splint every week!"

She also felt I'd done too much shot-gunning by trying different doctors. "Stick with one doctor only. Too much confuses the system."

"We *can* help you," she said, "It'll take a lot of care and a lot of work. A year at least once a week." (At $50 a twenty minute session--not to mention the cost of supplements.)

---

[1] Temple Mandibular Joint

The back pain was maddeningly intense--prickly pressure, very painful no matter what position I tried. Lying on my stomach was best. Everything in the house remained undone. Boxes and bags of books were strewn around the living room. Attending to tasks took too much energy.

Where will the money come from? When will this search end? I hated spending time and money on doctors when there was so much else I'd rather do. *Then why do I do it? Because I'm still looking for relief and resolution "Out There."*

> *"The Greeks did not even think about enjoying happiness without taking pain in their stride. Pain was the soul's experience of evolution."*
>
> *Ivan Illich,* ***Medical Nemesis***

Two days later I dragged myself up my front steps, miserably drained. I felt as if I'd run a marathon without having the pleasure of moving and sweating. Tears had welled up throughout the day--on Trish's massage table, at Steve's house, in the afternoon as I walked, and then at home, out they poured in racking sobs. I was utterly overwhelmed by my feelings of futility and sadness, turmoil and stuckness.

My head throbbed with hammering questions. *Am I "listening to my body" or am I being lazy? Am I releasing attachments to body vanity or am I becoming a slob? Am I resting and healing or am I being apathetic instead? Am I growing stronger from my withdrawal from people or am I creating further isolation? Am I breaking through barriers or behaving irresponsibly?*

When my body had first crashed in 1983, I had written a poem called *Confusion.* Now I found and re-read it. Surprise washed over me, for the poem was like a blueprint of my journey. Amazingly, something in me had known, so early on, that I was embarked on a path of metamorphosis. Reading the poem helped me remember that ***of course*** I was perplexed and uncertain, and to celebrate it! Confusion was an indicator of the growth and change and rebirth that I was undergoing.

CONFUSION

Confusion can be accepted
even welcomed when
we understand
its potential.

Confusion is a symptom of
a shaking up
a dying off
a rebirth--all
a creative process.

Old habits slough off new ones remain unformed
Old needs like old friends
no longer suffice
new ones are untested.

Rejoice in confusion, it
presages growth
creation
death
of that which must die.

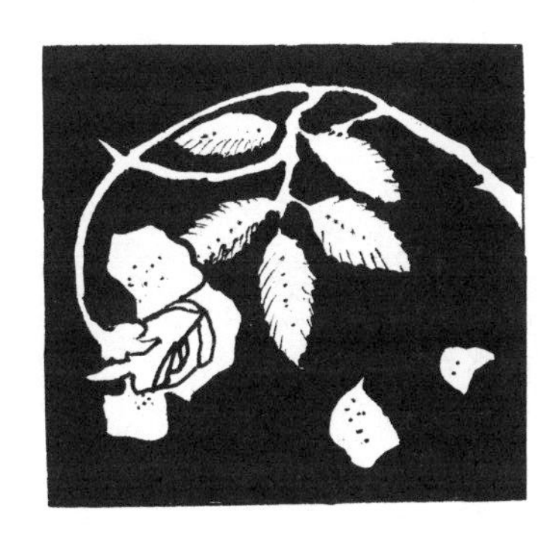

CHAPTER THIRTY-EIGHT

EVERY SO OFTEN, besides attending the Tuesday night classes, I'd have a private session with Mike Gotesman. In the course of one meeting, he said to me, "You're pushing the river. Trying too hard. You are pursuing healing and spirituality with the same tenacity and intensity that you put into your work."

"Can you relax? Can you just do a sauna in the sauna? No books or letters. Read when you're reading. Let your activity of the moment be pure. You'll find your energy is more focused and you'll have more of it."

Mike's simple admonishment was a turning point. Since that day I have applied this principle and found it to be very true. Of course I forget and sometimes race frantically about trying to accomplish several things at once. Then I immediately notice the frazzled energy and I can be sure that I don't accomplish nearly as much as when I do "pure" activity.

On another day I returned from doing errands and sank onto the couch thinking, *There'd be some hearty laughs if I shared what I've discovered ... that shopping can be a spiritual exercise.* I had started thinking differently about such daily drudgery things as cleaning and shopping. Instead of putting my life on hold and blitzing through errands and duties so that I could resume my "real" activities once I came home, I practiced the principles I was learning in Mike's class. When the salesgirl was new or slow, I practiced patience. I chose vegies and hunted for items, and waited in lines, just observing and letting it all unfold as it would. I asked myself, *What can I bring into this process, what gift can I give the checkout clerks, the other customers?* The answer was, *I give goodwill, smiles, calmness, patience, non-judgement, encouragement.* In this way I was being completely in the moment, letting the process, rather than hurrying home, be my goal.

How fortunate I felt to have the time to take for such activities--to be able to cultivate this way of being without the pressure of deadlines and obligations. Since I wasn't working or involved with a family, I wasn't focused on important responsibilities that would otherwise undermine my energy and interest in doing it.

At home a gallon jug of apple juice fell from the car and smashed in the driveway. Squatting in the rain sweeping it up, I thought about how the nature of glass, when it crashes into concrete, anyway, was to shatter. How perfectly the jug had fulfilled its nature. I took the time to notice each shard, each fragment, letting the process just be.

> *"If we do not choose suicide, how do we live in such a chaotic absurd, suffering world? The Hasidic commitment is to 'Joy in the world as it is, a life as it is, in every hour of life in this world as that hour is.' This means the hallowing of everyday life, taking each experience not as good or bad, but as natural ... accepting my feelings not because they are constructive or moral, or healthy, but simply because they are **mine**, **here**, and **now**."*
> *Sheldon Kopp,* ***If You Meet the Buddha on the Road Kill Him***

That night after class I eagerly hurried home to write and process. The session with Mike had generated an inner excitement as the concepts penetrated deeper and more convincingly. At home, I wrote lying on my stomach in the blue room. Betty Boop was propped like a nesting hen right between my legs, puttering away.

We had talked about the perfect meditation experience as being that time "when I am not there." I'd had such times when I was playing the piano or singing or writing. I'd finish and suddenly realize that I just spent half an hour or an hour writing, without thought to self. It might be that I was writing *about* self, but that didn't mean that I was aware of the self intruding into that moment.

In July when I massaged Dad in the convalescent home, I'd had the feeling of stepping aside. It was a time of just being. I'd felt "in my power." What I'd done was let go of the judging of the experience as being good or bad, and let it unfold from my heart.

Thinking back on the day and the evening as I lay in bed, I realized how perfect it has been. My time alone meditating, shopping, my time alone with the dishes, with the cats, reading, walking, my meeting with Mike.

It could be no other way, I mused. *I would be so contradictory if I was pursuing business or if I was putting energy into a relationship. I'd not be fully there. I am in my gestation period--developing and changing every day--sometimes hourly. Awarenesses alter and deepen. Insights follow one on the other. At the end of the week it is as if I've come, oh, so far--into another country--from the one in which I started at the beginning of the week.*

I began to acknowledge the positives in having my lessons come *not* as I would perceive or choose them. Who was I to presume that I could possibly know what was the way for me? Whenever I longed for my experiences to be a certain way, or to manifest like other people's, I was bound for disappointment. My lessons never appeared as I anticipated, and now I was beginning to see that that was right. They unfolded as they should be for me.

> *"There is no prescribed Way*
> *for everyone.*
> *There is just your Way for NOW--*
> *until you choose another."*
> *Rusty Berkus,* ***Appearances***

December 14th, my birthday, arrived. *Forty one. Truly an accomplishment.* The day before, at Mike's, he had said, "I sense something good and positive happening to you. It's going to be easier."

"Can you give me a clue?"

"I don't know what ..."

I thought how nice it would be to have some positive change after so many months of negativity and confusion. I could barely imagine that it could happen. The happiest thought I could conjure up was, *Maybe I'll have a good series of colonics.*

After leaving Mike's, I drove down to the Aspires graduation in Eugene. It was a fun, happy, heartful occasion. Diane O. kindly offered to let me sleep in her room in the Hilton. Thus my needs for the night were handled exactly as I'd fantasized. Diane and I bantered and joked in a delightful laugh-filled conversation, and it was two a.m. before we turned out the light. The next morning Diane requested that room service deliver our breakfast, and she wouldn't hear of my paying on my birthday.

Enter Diane, who participated in my PES, but until this point with whom I'd made only cursory contact. How could either of us guess the degree to which she would be one of the most important links in my life--or that I would one day live on her property on the Sandy River? With Diane, a Montessori School teacher, the child part of the personality is ever allowed to play, and she would be my teacher in many ways.

Back in Portland that evening, in honor of my birthday I treated myself to Rice Dream (non-dairy ice cream) for dessert. Alas, my healthy intentions foundered when I sprinkled on a little carob powder, a handful of raisins, and then a little more, and finally figured, *What the hell!* and doused it with Grand Marnier. Yummy. I devoured the whole pint.

> *"And I don't know what's coming,*
> *But this new day feels fine,*
> *My whole life is a poem,*
> *And the words and the rhythms are mine.*
> *Happy Birthday! Happy Birthday! Happy Birthday!"*
> *from,* ***I'm Getting My Act Together and Taking It on the Road***

Shortly after my birthday, a new course was introduced, one which I'd certainly not anticipated. On a cold, sunny morning I took several baskets of crystals to the Golden Butterfly New Age shop. Angus Thomas, the owner, happened also to be the past owner of the Portland Hypnosis Center. It hadn't been my thought when I went in, but I found myself saying, "I'm willing to trade crystals for hypnosis lessons."

Angus responded enthusiastically, saying, "I'll teach you the tools and the art of hypnosis. I promise that when we're done, you'll know enough to become certified."

What a turn of the tide. My next three months were to become punctuated by weekly hypnosis sessions with Angus. Not to mention that with his large order, I was actually getting back my investment in the crystals *plus* some profit!

The exciting and incredible thing was that a year before I wouldn't have traded anything. Operating out of a survival mode, I could only see the need for money. Now I found myself with a commodity--crystals--almost through no energy of my own (thanks to my dowsing friends), and having released my so-called need to trade for money, a completely new area of learning and experience had opened up for me.

A few days later I flew to California to spend Christmas with my family. Thankfully, my energy, though not terrific, was the best it had been in a long time. On my return trip to Portland, as I watched the landscape below dissolving from golds and browns into greens and purples, I reviewed my stay in Santa Cruz. I felt very complete, very satisfied with this parental visit. Originally I'd wished to avoid it, fearing the obstacles and doubting my ability to give to Mom and Dad. But now, sitting on the plane, I realized that, in truth, my presence did give them much. I also got much. I got their love, their vulnerability, their fear, their hope, their yearning. I got to share from my heart. Not in a gruff, blunt, dramatic way. Soft, gentle, "This is what's going on for me ... Let me show you how to cook this ... Your Minimum Hug Requirement is 12 per day ... See? You hold each other thus ... Let's try these exercises ... Great ... You're both doing so well ..."

I ate taboo foods--donuts, desserts, wheat, cheese, ice cream--and had fun doing it. None to excess. Just enough to taste, perhaps taste a second time, and then stop.

The idea began to grow that whatever money and health I had was there for me to use uplifting and giving to others. I felt that I was beginning to be able to emerge from my cocoon, and that part of my future "work" would be to fly to Santa Cruz to support and love and help Mom and Dad as often as I could.

It was four in the morning on the first day of the New Year. Despite my sleepiness, I decided to write. *With what portentous possibilities,* I wondered, *do I inscribe "1986?"* With what lushness my spirit was filled, brimming with the peace and warmth and welcome and love of the people who had filled my house that night.

I AM HOME. I've come home--home to Oregon, yes, and more. It's a daily returning. And I have no longer any question or doubts that I've found what I've been looking for: Wholeness in myself. Wholeness in others. The rightness and satisfaction of opening up to people, of offering the house, my food, my music, my ***self*** *to them. Creating a space in which individuals can be soft, gentle, loving of one another.*

Ahmad, uprooted at 60 from Iran, had beamed, "It's the best time I've had in America," and then he phoned me as soon as he got home to thank me again and to repeat that. Sweet, dear, little man. *How touched I am, and so glad that we met at the pool and that I invited you.*

Everyone commented about the warmth and the good feelings they had in my house. I had always thought that a party is what the participants themselves bring to it. I believed, after that night, however, that there is another piece--the atmosphere of warmth and welcome. I was happy to set the stage and share it. The bowls and swags of juniper and holly berries pungently permeated the room. No one had seen a tree with so many ornaments. The cats in their bright red bows totally accepted the people, lingering in their midst offering themselves to be picked up and handled.

Just before midnight we wrote down our "throw-away items" and thrust them into the flaming box of the wood stove. I wrote, *I throw away doctors and illness.* Then we were gently guided by Steve to close our eyes and meditate with a special focus on peace. We all sat quietly in the orange light of the fire and flickering candles, and after a few moments the haunting strains of *Pachabel Canon* stole across the silent room. Steve said, "Think about letting the year 1985 go and of going gracefully forward into 1986. Open your eyes on 1986."

Truly this year started out as I wanted. Not that I anticipated it. There's such a sense of peace and calm and accepting and trusting. I've found it in myself, and in each person here, in Mom and Dad and Sis, and in the ripple that we each send out into the world. In giving a place of welcome to Ahmad and Janish and all the others, I give myself welcome.

And now--so much to look forward to. How would it evolve? The psychic had commented, "Your health is improving." Mike had said, "Something good is going to happen." The artist lady who sees visions told me, "There is hope, rejuvenation, brightness in the spring." John Honse predicted, "In March or April your life will stand on its head." *I want to be ready! I want to look good! Such vanity.*

> *"... you have progressed far enough to feel a measure of safety, of surety in your position. Now, it is time to turn again and face the future reassured and prepared to share the good fortune that comes."*
>
> *The Rune of Movement, from* ***The Book of Runes***

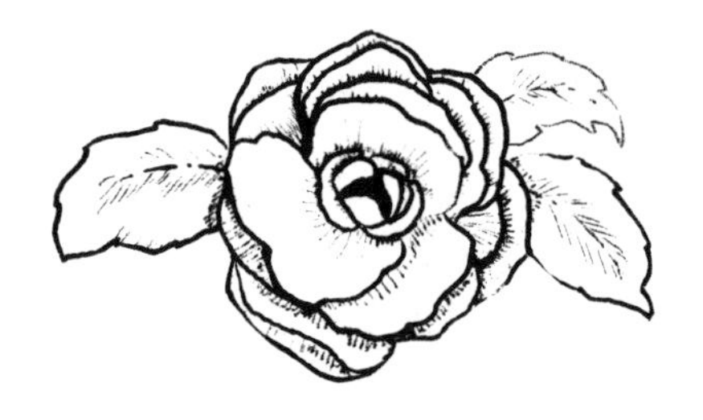

PART VI

WATCH FOR SIGNS OF SPRING

Remember the seed of the new is present in the shell of the old. The new seed is the seed of unrealized potential, a seed of good. Your present conduct will either bring the new fruit to ripeness or cause it to rot on the vine. You must trust your own process and watch for signs of spring.

The Rune of Initiation, from ***The Book of Runes***

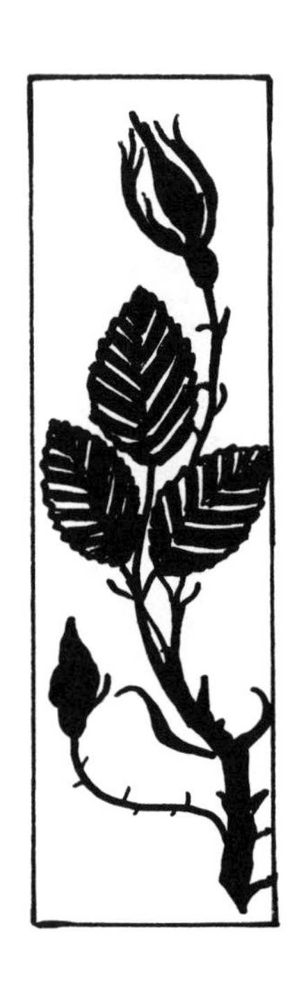

CHAPTER THIRTY-NINE

IT WAS JANUARY fourth, a glittering, cold and frosty day. Two letters arrived from Santa Cruz, one from Dad and one from Mom. Pretty special as neither had written for months. Throughout the day my thoughts flitted back to those letters, and I felt warmed, contented, so pleased that I'd followed my heart and taken risks.

The letters were a validation that my Santa Cruz trip at Christmas *had* been a success, that I *had* reached my parents in the way I'd wanted to. Dad's letter, unlike recent conversations and previous letters, was full of life, written in a strong hand, and even expressed interest and involvement in daily affairs. The most incredible part of the short note, though, was that he signed it "with lots of love, Dad." How that brief line stirred my spirit and my heart. He'd never been that direct or effusive. I believed that, indeed, my presence really had made a difference.

Before going to Santa Cruz I had thought that I'd resolved all I wanted to with my parents. Yet the Christmas together revealed that there were further steps to be taken--steps of which I'd had no inkling. We had crossed boundaries that I'd stopped at before. Now I wondered what further undreamed of connections I might be able to facilitate through future letters and visits. I also wondered, *Could I have ever affected this outreach and this bonding if I'd not undergone these last two years?*

Because of my willingness to risk, stretch, and give, from that time and during the next two years until their deaths, my relationship with my parents blossomed beyond what I'd have imagined possible. It was a continually deepening process teaching me that there were always further possibilities if I would but open to them.

At Aspires the following morning, so many people spontaneously commented, "You're looking good," that I began to wonder how "bad" I used to look. When I was at my lowest ebb, how drained and ill must I have appeared? Even more strange was the fact that in recent months I had inexorably gained weight. *How can it be*, I wondered, *that 15 more pounds--weighing 130!!!--has not had the effect of making me look "worse?"* I remembered Antoine de Saint-Exupery's statement in *The Little Prince, "It is only with the heart that one can see rightly: what is essential is invisible to the eye,"* and thought, *It must apply to what people are seeing in me.*

That afternoon Victor phoned. Would I be willing to organize and conduct some cooking and candida classes for the Whole Health Center? Although I was reluctant to involve myself with a workaday routine I thought, *This will be a good stretch, and it will bring in some money.* So I agreed. As soon as I hung up the receiver, I picked it up again and initiated the process of researching and scheduling places, dates, printers, flyers. The sap was rising. It felt good to be productive. It also felt scary. My thoughts began to charge about, and my stomach tightened up as I entered into the pressure of organizing and being responsible and having it all come out "right."

I'm dipping my toe into the mainstream of the everyday world and, like cold water, it's a shock to my system. The key is to know that it will come out "right" no matter how it comes out. Some wise part of me ***knows****, so I don't have to struggle, don't have to do anything. That part, which Steve calls the "Big I," is handling it all. I simply have to shut up, slow down, and get out of my way.*

Two nights later I went out to dinner with my Iranian friend, Ahmad. At the end of the evening, I said goodbye to him in front of his apartment. As I steered my car into the street, I looked back at Ahmad standing alone in the dark driveway. He stood, a slight, erect little man with bandy legs, his wool hat in his hand held over his heart. He lifted the other hand in a last wave as I backed up my car and then turned into the street to drive home. My heart stirred, and I felt the tears welling. His presence had touched me. He called me his daughter, "better than a niece." He was a sweet, dear man who believed in giving to his children and who would give to all if he could.

And now he was returning to whatever fate awaited him in Iran.

Would the revolutionary government refuse to honor his pension and his assets? Would they throw him in jail for his past association with the Shah? Would his reputation serve to keep him safe? My heart went out to him. He wanted to serve, to be useful, to give, and he could see only that Iran was the place where he had the means to survive. He believed that he must either run a business or be a lawyer--that he couldn't do other things like tutoring students or managing apartments. He'd bought a restaurant, which failed miserably, and in the course of nine years he went through all the money he had brought with him from Iran. His divorce took more than money from him. The children listened to the mother and didn't understand his situation.

At the restaurant that night he told me these things so matter of factly. Then, eyes twinkling, he would make some bright remark or joke. As we bantered and laughed together his face crinkled all over in a big smile.

Tonight was spiritual, I thought to myself. *Barbara got out of the way. She let the "Big I" run the show, and it was perfect, of course.* I had even resolutely resisted the urge to check my watch so that I could be home for the Agatha Christie movie at nine o'clock. I had let everything flow as it would and found myself surprised at how easily conversation flowed, at how much I found to talk about with Ahmad.

When I deposited Ahmad at his apartment I had given him a crystal and a little note of bon voyage. Then I drove home, deeply moved by this brave little man, and by the connection of one self with another. And I got home exactly in time for the nine o'clock movie!

A week after I said goodbye to Ahmad, my final divorce papers arrived in the mail. It was official. A completion. Jack and I were no longer man and wife in the eyes of the law. I phoned Jack and wished him, "Happy divorce. It was nice going through it with you."

He said, "I can't think of anyone I'd rather have done it with."

The mail that day had been good to me. Besides two letters from Australia, my postbox also gave forth a letter from my mother. Her back was feeling better since she started doing the exercises I showed her at Christmas. She and Dad had started attending the senior citizen lunches and were enjoying them. She wrote, "Your last letter was like a wise lecture."

I must surprise them with my "wisdom," I thought, *And I am prepared now to keep revealing it, to let go of my fears and excuses for holding myself back. The outcome I want with Mom and Dad is connection. I've opened to sharing love and hugs with all the other people around me. That is who I am now. I want to do the same with my parents.* We had come a long way, and I held to the hope that, with time, my parents could increasingly relax their fears about showing their emotions and uninhibitedly express their love and hug me back.

As part of my program toward being better able to give to others, I decided to learn how to give massages. John Honse was also interested, so he and I began weekly lessons with Peter. I came home from the first session as high as a kite. The hour had started with John on the table and my mimicking the strokes and movements that Peter demonstrated. I felt no residue of Peter's and my old relationship. Just pleasure in the friendship and the learning. I felt strong and sure and confident of my ability and enjoyed the process. Enjoyed the movement of my hands on skin and muscles, the assimilating of all the skills I could bring to affect the well-being of the body's tissues.

For the first time I experienced what tense muscle tissue felt like and could feel the hardened deposits in a person's organs. Massage drew me--as a way to give more than the skills of my hands to somebody. It also reflected something Steve had said to me, "When you give of yourself, through massage or otherwise of your own health, you are demonstrating that you have health to give."

> *"How much are you willing to give?"*
> *Rusty Berkus,* ***Appearances***

Despite the highs of the morning massage lesson, my mood slid into melancholy later that afternoon. Bundled up against the bitter cold, I forged out along the winding streets and paths of my neighborhood loop. Yet again, for the third winter, I approached the little tree in the park. It was the first blooming tree of the season, and each year I was attracted to its manifestation of life's renewal. It was the scraggliest of trees, yet its survival and fruition amidst its larger cousins commanded my respect and appreciation.

Each year I had been telling myself: *I, too, am renewing. I, too, am budding. I, too, will blossom in the spring and flourish in the summer.* And each winter I came back, walking heavily as I had the year before, and wondered, *Will this be the year in which I will come dancing and running into the park?*

Two weeks later my energies were "up." It was late afternoon and I sat on the living room floor with three little chips lined up in front of me. This was my first effort at reading a Rune spread, and it catapulted me into a "wow" experience. Earlier that morning I had bought the Rune book and the little velvet bag containing chips with hieroglyphs on them. Whenever I'd done a workshop with Steve, or when he'd given me a Rune quote at our counselling sessions, the oracles had seemed so right for that moment. Now I smiled, awed by the message presented by the Runes which my hand had drawn forth from the burgundy colored bag.

"*The problem,*" they said, "*is to cleanse, realign, and reevaluate, to keep letting go of the old ruts, habits, thoughts that hold you back. Persevere. The harvest is indeed coming. Be assured and be patient. It comes not in your pushing or pulling, but will come in the perfect time.*"

How encouraging! There was a note of certainty as I said to myself, *I **am** healing and growing and finding that inner wholeness. I **know** the harvest is coming.*

In the evening after dinner, it felt right to leave the warm house and fire, don boots and layers of warm clothes, and walk in the late season snow flurries. I loved the fantasy they created. The world seemed exquisitely new and magical whenever snow arrived. I was drawn, as ever, to the park. I *ran* across the lawn, retextured now with snow, to my noble little tree. Standing beneath it and the circle of other mighty trees, I lifted my arms, and said, *Hello!*

High up at their peaks, the trees gently nodded. They stood, drawn up in the dark, protective, their branches tiered like ballerinas' ball gowns sweeping the ground. Behind their silhouettes the sky was creamy charcoal-pink and snow flakes fell in peaceful silent shadows all around.

Truly there is some strong change in my body, I said, aloud. I was feeling gloriously alert and energetic at this late hour and had been all day, in spite of the Aspires early morning and an interrupted sleep the previous night. And the same energy had been there the Tuesday before. Smiling, I told the trees, *I feel the momentum of "something" unfolding.*

A week later I was hurtling forward in a momentum of another kind. At six p.m. I would be conducting my first candida class at the Whole Health Center. Throughout the day, as I prepared for the evening, I was wound up, full of pulsing energy--and a good deal of nervousness. Finally I took a moment to sit quietly. Focusing on the nervousness, I created an image of it in my mind's eye. I imagined that the nervousness was a little "bundle" which I gently took from my head and placed outside myself. Feeling calmer, I asked myself, *What's the nervousness about?* The answer came, *It's about looking good, about giving the people value, about not failing.*

I'd read somewhere that before every undertaking we should take a moment to turn within, to open to letting the "Big I" flow in the enterprise. I was increasingly practicing this and it seemed to work, to fit, to feel right. I did this now.

Not surprisingly, my nervousness turned out to be for naught. The class went extremely well. I was totally relaxed. Briefly, at the beginning, I didn't have my stride, and then I hit it. Later, when I looked back on it, I recognized that as being the point where Barbara stepped out of the way.

The class was comprised of three single women and one woman with her husband, a good group to begin with. All had terrific histories of allergies and candida. All were stimulated to ask questions and I felt totally comfortable answering. Later, as I sat at home reviewing the evening, I chuckled. Mike had once said to our class, "You'll know when something is right. It flows. It just doesn't have the obstacles that are there when it's not right." This night had flowed.

Let me recognize that this **is** *what happened,* I urged myself. *Let me not discount it.* And I couldn't discount it! The entire evening progressed in a way that I'd rarely experienced when I'd led other groups. Smooth, easy, natural, comfortable. Fun! Not a burden or a big responsibility, not me concerned that people were getting or not getting whatever ... no thought about outcome. I was in the moment.

> *"The man who is flying beautifully does not think about landing. He knows it is the flying that is important, not arriving at the airfield or even returning to earth. He has transcended himself and has put himself in touch with the infinite."*
>
> *David Smith,* ***Healing Journey***

CHAPTER FORTY

IN AN EFFORT to transcend my distracting habits, I tried something I'd never before done. Although I related to no religious organizations, I felt that a place of retreat would help me get out of my own way. At Portland's Franciscan Renewal Center I did just that. In my five days there I delved deep, supported by the peace of the place. As I processed and as insights came, I filled three notebooks. The extracts that follow are tiny glimpses of this retreat experience.

10:00 a.m., February 13
Franciscan Renewal Center

I arrived in the silence of the blanketing snow, and now I sit in my airy nun's room. I start to unpack, but stop. No, I must open to the "Big I" guiding this enterprise. I sit on the narrow bed briefly, letting whatever comes, come. Here I am at the beginning. Or at the end?

What do I do? Do I employ discipline? Do I flow with my feelings? I feel sleepy. I am here to do inner work, but I hesitate to embark on it. It's akin to laying out a new project like painting. The materials are in their places. The goal is understood. There's that part, though, that hangs back, knowing it's going to be up to its elbows in paint and grit. That it won't be easy to come up for air, to stop for the phone, or to attend elsewhere once the hands are covered in paint. Yet I have nothing to distract me now. So---plunge in!

8:30 p.m.

Back in my little nook, the middle conference cubicle, warm and toasty, satisfied from dinner. I ate in the retreatants' dining room, whose carpet and Queen Anne furniture contrast softly with the institutional cafeteria. That room is much more in keeping with the flavor of the warm personal solitudinal atmosphere I want to steep in.

We eat in silence, the three of us. At first it seems awkward. The desire is to put forth the personality, to puppet the smiles and questions, the gestures that we've been trained to do. But we sit and eat, each in our own inner place, and I am thankful that I do not have to interrupt the flow of inner opening that was started this afternoon. I taste, taste, chew, chew, lift, lift, swallow, grateful to be excused from the rites of human interaction. "Keep thy mind staid upon me."

> *"Monastic life, as I see it, is a means of jettisoning bit by painful bit unnecessary "baggage," so that, getting progressively lighter, one's pace becomes correspondingly swifter. In themselves the monastic life and its traditions held no attraction for me. That they were all means to an end was something of which I was keenly aware."*
>
> *Mary O'Hara,* ***The Scent of Roses***

February 14
Franciscan Renewal Center

I glow in the awareness of the rightness of deciding to come to this retreat center, so perfect for me now. All is designed to support the retreatant in pursuing his/her path in whatever way they choose. I don't have to exchange small talk or life histories. I don't have to worry about planning, eating, or even attending meals. The snack rooms amply accommodate me should I decide that I don't want to interrupt wherever I'm at to go to eat.

I read and meditate, walk, read and meditate, and "Keep my mind stayed on God," and I find it easy to do. It has nothing to do with having visions or seeing lights or hearing voices or any of those outer images that we all love to learn about and wish to emulate.

It is *my* inward journey, *my* deepening awareness of the spiritual consciousness within me. I accept what comes, knowing that each step is one more piece of the way which only I can walk. Whose city do I wind up in if I follow another man's path?

> *"Each of us has a unique predicament that requires a unique journey."*
>
> *Ram Dass*

February 15
Franciscan Renewal Center

Dinner. Silent. There are five of us tonight in the quiet dining room. How I appreciate this way of being alone. Out in the main dining room a group of men and women guests have arrived. We retreatants serve up our food along with them. The noise of conversation sounds strange, especially with the bass of men's voices. I also find the presence of men jarring. I've liked not taking thought of hair, face, clothes, or personal interactions. Here are the men, and I notice that a new element is introduced.

After dinner I spontaneously decide that I'd like to do a Rune for relationships with men. Relationships seem so remote, so far from my need or desire. The Rune that comes up is: Standstill. That which impedes. Ice. This Rune signifies that I am in a winter period. Patience (How often that word comes up!). This fallow period, in fact, precedes a rebirth (That word too!) There's a freeze on useful activity, all plans are on hold. Energy feels an unaccustomed drain because of the chill wind that blows over me from the ice floes of old outmoded habits. I must let go, shed, release, cleanse away the old. That will bring on the thaw.

This describes my whole life, as well as relationships. It seems that the character of the last three years has been that of one big enema. A constant push to let go and eliminate the old habits and beliefs that created the illness in the first place. I truly trust that the thaw is coming. I feel it.

February 16
Franciscan Renewal Center

I cannot hurry the germination process. I cannot force the shoots up, cannot push the baby down the birth canal before it is ready. I can recognize that this is where I am in the process--can relax and enjoy the moments that comprise it. Why not have fun and be light with it? Must creation and birth be so solemn?

> *"Does one really have to fret*
> *About enlightenment?*
> *No matter what road I travel,*
> *I'm going home."*
> *Shinsho, in Ram Dass's* ***Journey of Awakening***

8:00 p.m.

I sat for hours in the chapel. It felt right to be there, quiet, intense, if that word can be applied to meditation. This afternoon as I meditated I asked inside, *What must I leave behind?*

What came to me was: *Everything. You can take nothing with you.*

Everything!?

Tonight I again ask, *Everything? How can I leave everything behind. I'm afraid.*

You must leave your fears behind.

How?

Confront your fears.

Anxiety swarms over me. How can I possibly confront all my fears and survive? The point is--living *with* fears is death. It is *not* surviving. The only way *anyone* survives, or truly lives, is by facing up to their fears. Fears are examples of "Nothing is good or bad but thinking makes it so." They are nothing more than my imaginings. And therefore they don't exist!

What ways do I confront fears? Being honest with Mom and Dad, plunging into ice cold rivers, giving money away instead of clinging to it, giving food away instead of hoarding it, giving clothes away instead of hanging on to them, setting my alarm for early morning instead of trying to squeeze another shred of sleep out of the night, stopping depending on pills and doctors instead of turning inside to my *own* healing powers, fasting, firewalking, jumping out of airplanes ...

I might screw up. I might die. Yet I know the opposite is true. That I am essentially dead as long as I don't dispense with these fears. As long as I refuse to deal with them I will continue to be a shell, unable to act. I must do another firewalk! How ridiculous that I can fear it, having already completed one.

Yuk. Yuk. Yuk. This is not the turn of events I would have chosen. Certainly not what the *body* would have chosen. I've just directed all this energy of the last two years into pursuing ways to support and preserve and heal this body, and now I tell it, "You're going to jump out of airplanes!"

In bed, feeling as if I've done deep work today. I'm exhausted emotionally. My sense is of having gone out to work on the drain pipes but of winding up slogging through the sewers instead.

February 17

Thomas Merton's words are so appropriate this morning: Why should I worry about losing a bodily life, that I must invariably lose anyway, as long as I possess a spiritual life and identity that cannot be lost? Why should I fear to cease to be what I am not ...?

> *"The unreal never is: the Real never is not ... Beyond the power of sword and fire, beyond the power of waters and winds, the Spirit is everlasting, omnipresent, never-changing, never-moving, ever One. Invisible is he to mortal eyes, beyond thought and beyond change. Know that he is, and cease from sorrow."*
>
> ***Bhagavad Gita***, *2:16-25*

February 18

I walk out of the convent almost in a trance. Driving home, the roads, the cars, the lights all look so foreign, so removed. At home I greet the kits and then walk in the dark park, remembering the lyrics to *The Rose*. Last June in PES I sang *The Rose*. The song is about me. Like the Runes and the psychics and the astrology chart, *The Rose* reassures me that there *is* a spring. I'm now in my winter, and ever more aware of the degree of my isolation and of wanting to have connection. I know the seed of love is germinating within. When will be my spring?

"Just remember in the winter,
Far beneath the bitter snows,
Lies the seed that with the sun's love,
In the spring becomes the Rose."
from, ***The Rose***

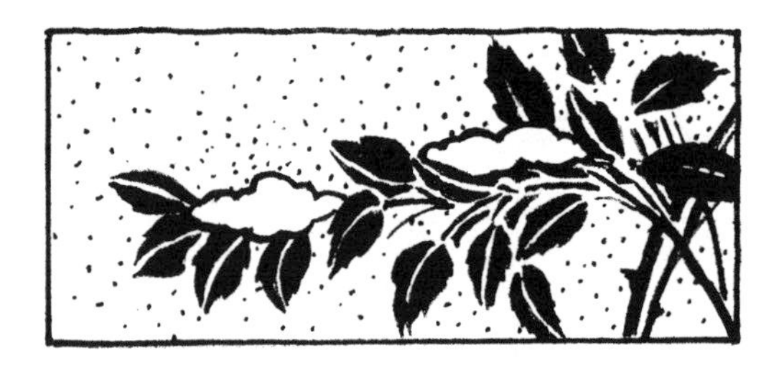

CHAPTER FORTY-ONE

IN THE WEEKS following my retreat at the Franciscan Renewal Center, everywhere I went I offered free massages to friends. I wanted to practice massage *and* overcome fears. And every so often this little smile raised itself inside me. It was related to the budding awareness that was developing regarding work. The idea was such a foreign one that it only cropped up occasionally and then it was gone as soon as I recognized it. There had come these flickerings of realization that: *Life is* ***fun****. Life is* ***easy****.* My being could barely recognize such a concept, let alone accept it. And so this little smiling light danced away. Then, perhaps a day later, it danced back into and over my imagination for another brief moment.

It was this incredible idea that I truly could make a living, earn an income, do some work, have a social life ... *and* it could be enjoyable, easy, fun. The activities that were evolving--the crystals, the massage, the classes, were all doing so in such a non-stressful, unpressured way.

I loved staying at home and having massage or candida clients drop in. Loved the idea of hosting cooking or crystal evenings in my house and started planning for them. Rather than anticipating that these activities would bring struggles, obstacles, and pressure, it began to occur to me that nothing had to change. My life could continue in its calm way *and* I could be earning an income or studying too.

I couldn't help but wonder if I was in self-deception. Could it really be this simple? *And why not?* I asked myself. *It will be nice to let go of the old concept of life as struggle once and for all.*

> *"... strugglers like to feel that struggle is noble--that somehow God is pleased with them for struggling. If you were God, you would fall over laughing at that one."*
>
> *Stuart Wilde,* ***Life Was Never Meant to be a Struggle***

At the end of February an opportunity arose for me to bring more of my issues into focus. I had been preparing, through a course of several weekly trainings, to assist on a back-up team in the Wings seminars. The back-up team members played crucial roles in assisting the seminar participants as well as the facilitators. Not only did the team members learn and grow through serving others, but the situations that came up put them in line for a personal development experience which was akin to that of being once again a seminar participant.

On my second day as a back-up team member of the PES, I was standing in the back of the large room listening to the trainer address the group. I thought how we were like a company of passengers gathered on a cruise ship for five days. All present were committed to this particular journey and were active within the boundaries of this unique world. All externals were left behind.

I had found that the cruise, for me, was a totally new PES experience. I'd changed so much, had come so far, since being a participant eight months earlier. Also, as a back-up team member, I was on the training side of the fence. I'd felt trepidation about tackling some of the tasks which were given to me, particularly that of leading the Small Circle Feedback. Once I plunged into the process, however, it flowed smoothly. I had a maternal, protective, nurturing feeling toward my group of five. In the feedback they gave me, they said they saw me as "serene, calm, digesting words before I commented--" *Wouldn't they be amazed if they could have seen me in the PES last June!*

I was moved by the moving my people were doing. By the end of the second day, Tim, the older man whom I'd at first resisted, let tears fall as we did the closing feedback. My appreciation grew, too, for certain fellow team members, especially Andre. He reminded me of Alan, another deceptively young, short man, surprise package, full of integrity and expressing himself clearly and compassionately.

As I drove home at midnight after this second day, I had the feeling of being about to bust loose--like a big slab of rock was being pried off me with a crowbar. *When that rock finally flies off,* I told myself, *I will be free, will be truly me, and that enthusiasm, love, fun, wisdom, and so much that I only glimpse now, will flow, will dance me into the world.*

> *"All earthly pain*
> *is due to our inability to*
> *release what needs to be free.*
>
> *When you release*
> *what needs to be free,*
> *YOU are freed in the process."*
> *Rusty Berkus,* ***Appearances***

In the course of the PES week, I confronted and wrestled with several personal issues, the biggest one being that of learning to trust myself in the moment, of being able to act without planning ahead. Another issue that burgeoned into full focus was that of how I interacted with strong, powerful people. Watching myself relate to the seminar trainers during the week I saw the boundaries I'd set up for myself. Around the mild and meek I seemed to be "me." Around the strong and powerful I went into comparison, assuming that I was unacceptable to them at their level. The kind of people that I wanted in my life were the very ones from whom I held myself back.

Putting myself in the seminar had been a step in the direction of addressing this issue. Help came, too, from talking with dear Peter, ever my mentor, on the day after the PES ended. Peter's questions and comments helped direct me toward the answers within.

"You've been in this pool where the people around you are soft, wonderful people but are also not especially dynamic and powerful. You provide strength, support and insight, but when *you* need support, the dynamics are not drawn up that way. Failing to get the intimacy you need, you're starving for that level of relationship."

I was suddenly aware that it was the equivalent of depriving myself of nourishment if I deprived myself of dynamic and stimulating people. *No wonder I eat and eat hoping to be fulfilled and that I seek tasty foods that will give me stimulation.* I simply could no longer choose malnourishment. It was like suddenly discovering that I needed protein in the diet. I would certainly remedy that lack.

A leap was being made--the leap from being afraid of intruding on others to accepting, more surely than ever before, that I was indeed giving. *The desire is to give,* I told myself, *to no longer hide my talents, and "to dare to give them away." (Each Day a New Beginning) The isolation I've accepted is appropriate no more.*

My blossoming confidence was reflected in my sessions with Steve Hillinger. They were taking on a different texture, becoming more of an interchange of equals rather than a guiding of one advanced being to a lessor one. Certainly, I did come for guidance and growth. Now, though, I recognized that I gave the same to Steve in different ways.

One morning I expressed this to him, telling him how I was opening up to being with "equal" or "advanced" people without apology, without holding back. I found myself saying, "I have gifts and teachings flowing through me that even you can learn from."

He smiled and nodded, "That's true."

"I'm beginning to realize that it's actually detrimental to my well-being when I'm behaving as if my offerings are not good enough."

"And you know what's even *worse*?"

I shook my head.

"When you hold back. Because then you rip me off. You deny me the things that I can learn from you."

The day after the session with Steve was a landmark. I had offered to give my friend, Ellen, a massage. Everything went well and I got into a nice rhythm once I stopped *thinking* about what I should or should not be doing. The massage was supposed to be free, but Ellen paid me $15 anyway, brightly saying, "This is your tip!" Immediately after she'd left, I hurried into the office and made a file for MASSAGE INCOME. Smiling with pleasure, I entered: *March 15: $15.*

A few days later I gave another friend a massage. Afterward, we drank tea together and she commented, "You seem like a different person than the one I met at Victor's ten months ago. I thought you were kind of a lightweight. Now there's a sort of elegance."

Interestingly, at Mike's class the previous Tuesday, Susan had said to me, "I don't know what it is, but your face is different."

There *was* a difference in my face. I could see it too. I liked it better. It wasn't so askew. It was more lined up. *The result of the TMJ splint?* I wondered. *But there's that calm, too, that I don't ever remember. And yes, I agree, an elegance. Is it the reflection of my inner self?*

Even so, I was still stuck in comparison. I couldn't imagine what it would be like to just be with people--women especially--and not measure myself against them. I only did this with women who were a certain way--attractive, assured, extroverted, successful.

"Upon an ordinary material thing we can look with reverence, wondering simply at its being. But when we look upon a human face, we interpret it by what we are ourselves. And what are we?"

Iris Murdock, ***The Sandcastle***

The end of March was approaching. People bought crystals and dropped by for massages. The money and abundance and people were flowing. I was very conscious of the gifts funnelling through me and that they were for me to share. Oddly, I did not fear that if I did this I would lack in any way. Instead, there was an absolute rightness about following my heart, my inner voice--if that was it--urging me to flow outward, give outward. I was putting aside fears of not being good, clever, or advanced enough, healthy or wealthy enough. *People benefit from my gifts.* ***I*** *benefit from them.*

"... ask yourself and yourself alone one question. It is this: "Does this path have a heart?" All paths are the same. They lead nowhere. They are paths going through the brush or into the brush or under the brush. Does this path have a heart is the only question. If it does, then the path is good. If it doesn't, it is of no use."

Carlos Castanada, ***The Teachings of Don Juan***

CHAPTER FORTY-TWO

BENEATH THE SURFACE of my days there was an underlying current--of something building. I could feel the change coming. SOMETHING. I went about my activities, though, focused in the moment as best I could, keeping expectations low-key. I attended Mike's class, gave massages, walked, wrote, had times together with friends. I booked a flight to Santa Cruz for April, not hesitating to buy the ticket, but inwardly realizing that this plan might very well change. I felt that the passage of the last three years and the acceleration of these past six months, had been aimed at getting me to some coming moment.

One of the activities which kept me focused in the present was another firewalk. Steve had asked me to participate in a demonstration at OMSI (Oregon Museum of Science and Industry) as part of an Indian exhibit.

The morning of the walk I awakened early, wondering, *What will Barbara do? Will she get out of the way*? Inside a voice had said, *This is to be fun, NOT SERIOUS*. I looked around in wonder and thought, *Why not?*

At noon I joined Steve and his assistant, Susan, at OMSI. The outdoor fire area was cordoned off and attracted many people from the milling crowds wandering about the nearby pavilion. We three waited, sitting or standing, mostly in silence, for the fire to burn down.

Originally, I felt very centered, with no real doubt about walking. When the crowd began to gather, however, the body started calling attention to itself, doing its nervous thing, heart pounding, legs shaking. Only then did I begin to question, *Can I do this without the "ideal" conditions, without the usual centering exercises that prepare us? Can I do this with so much nervousness?*

Steve gathered me and Susan under each arm and said, "Okay, team ..." and started walking us toward the fire. Looking at me, he said, "This might be a sign for you to learn that you can do things any time ... since an issue for you is fearing that you're not ready or prepared enough, don't have enough education, not good enough ..."

What a stretch. The crowd seemed to display a side-show mentality about the firewalk. Joking and laughter filled the air. Yet when my turn came, after Steve and Susan had each walked, I stood still, gathering my inner calm. Staring at the coals, I didn't wonder *if* I would walk. I just wondered *when.* I forgot the crowd. My heart pounded and my stomach twisted in knots. I walked. People clapped. Susan gave me a hug. Relief. And still turmoil. *Should I walk again?* I wanted to, yet ...

After Steve walked once more, the crowd dispersed. Many people approached us and asked questions. An interviewer from the *Oregonian* took notes. "What does it do for you?" he asked me.

"I confront fear in a different way." I spoke of the opportunity that this particular experience had been, "I'd entertained a belief that I needed certain supportive conditions in order to do a firewalk--and other things in my life--and today's experience just proved that it's only a belief."

> *"How can you come to know yourself? Never by thinking; always by doing. Try to do your duty, and you'll know right away what you amount to. And what is your duty? Whatever the day calls for."*
>
> *Goethe, from* ***Hatha Yoga*** *by Kathleen Hitchcock*

At the beginning of the week, Sis phoned and brought me up to date on the family news. She told me about Mom's surprise birthday party, about the new car that was on order, Dad's improvement. Before she could hang up, I asked, "Did Mom and Dad mention that I was firewalking on Sunday?"

"No."

"Did they ever mention that I firewalked last spring?"

"No."

"Well, goodbye."

I seemed bereft of receiving any recognition from my family. And there was no one around who offered it. Although I told myself that it wasn't that important, I couldn't help feeling isolated from human supporters. It seemed that there was no one to whom I could turn who would understand or acknowledge the achievement of my survival, of my growth, of my hunger for growth. Steve kept his comments very non-committal. At least, though, I could express things to him.

The next night, Marc, from Mike's class, came for his free massage. His feedback was kindly put. "It feels like you're playing my foot like a piano ... Your hands are caring ... You have passion in your hands ... As you get practice, the rest will come. You'll begin to notice what each body is calling for. You'll get the feel. It was wonderful!"

Marc struck me as an absolutely sweet man. I felt a strong attraction toward both him and his wife, Cathy, and felt so welcomed by them. After he had left, I sat on the couch smiling to myself. *I **am** starting to venture deeper into involvement with people whom I aspire to be like or with.* Betty snuggled into my lap. As I stroked her fur, I said, *See, Booper, things **are** looking up. I am continually learning the lesson that I **am** good enough. I **am** the vehicle for gifts which I bring to others. I **am** an enhancement to them. The diminishment occurs when I don't let myself be known.*

> *"You stand outside the circle*
> *and wonder why you feel left out,*
> *unaware that you need your OWN permission*
> *to join the others--*
> *not theirs."*
>
> *Rusty Berkus, **Appearances***

The following day was Saturday and I felt so good and my stomach looked so flat that I phoned Karl and invited him up for a roll in the sack. My timing was a bit off the mark. His parish priest and his sister, the nun, were visiting. He said, "I'll call you back later."

I redirected my energy from Karl to sweeping, cleaning, and

reading Ernest Gann's autobiography, *Hostage To Fortune.* It abounded with adventure and dynamism, risk-taking and audacity and what I once would have called amazing good luck. Now I saw luck differently. I recognized "luck" as Gann's level of openness to WHATEVER, which manifested in such forms as a job offer here or a serendipitous meeting there. *As I open myself to the revealing of my own inner self, I realize that I, too, contain within me that capacity for harmony, adventure, excitement, and the connection with stimulating and evolved people.*

A few days later I went to Trish for a massage but, instead, I gave her one. She was low, having been through a lot of turmoil and worry with her son's illness, and I was delighted to have something really worthwhile to give her. The massage allowed me to connect with her in a nonverbal way, giving her love, nurturing, relaxation and support through the touch of my hands. She loved it and repeatedly commented, "You're really good." She even said, "I don't think you need any more study!"

That's the way I felt as well. I already was able to give a credible massage from what I'd learned to date. I wondered, *Where am I going with massage? Will it be my work?* The awareness was growing that I truly need not "take thought," that the "Big I" was directing my life--perfectly.

I had been thinking a lot lately about the concepts of work and income. What were they, really? All my life I'd accepted the belief that declared that work should be something one is reimbursed for. With the internal changes that were taking place, though, I had begun to look at "work" differently. Throughout the last year, I had asked myself, *How should I earn a living? How can I do what I want* ***and*** *earn an income?* Now I realized, *Silly woman! Notice! For the last six months you've* ***done*** *what you wanted and you've been well supplied. The income--or supply--doesn't necessarily have to come from the work!*

WORK AND SUPPLY ARE NOT RELATED! WOW! This was dumbfounding--a breathtaking revelation. It was strange that I'd not seen it before, considering my flower business experience. In those days, the amount of income, or supply, had been totally unrelated to my slaving 16 hour days. *Something bigger than myself is the source of my supply. It manifests in all kinds of ways: in my walnut tree providing me and the squirrels with nuts, in the sun warming both me and the tree, in the dowser from Arkansas sending me crystals, and in Angus coming along and trading me hypnosis lessons for them.*

At the moment, my supply was coming to me in the *form* of the family money. It enabled me to do the giving I was doing. *And **that** is my work,* I thought, with a grin of recognition. *I've already found it. I've been doing it all along!*

It seemed so clear: *The gifts that flow through me are meant to **give**. The massage, the cooking, the talking and supporting and sharing ... is this not my "work?" I am learning to "take no thought" for supply or work. Both are supplied in whatever form the "Big I" chooses.*

How narrow I had been!--always looking only at how I could derive income from my labor. *At some inner level, every one of us lives in abundance, in infinite supply, in harmony,* I realized. *And we need never believe that our supply comes **only** from work. Certainly nature is an example of that. Supply comes. Supply **IS**.*

I was throbbing with excitement. Everything seemed crystal clear. I easily knew what to do about massage school and Cross Over back-up teams and about giving my time for various things. Follow my heart--my bliss. Let it flow. I certainly didn't need to study anatomy *per se*. The process for me was to simply deepen my ability to reach people in the ways that felt right for me, and to give, or "work," through every means that opened to me.

> *"... if you do follow your bliss you put yourself on a kind of track that has been there all the while, waiting for you, and the life that you ought to be living is the one you are living. When you can see that, you begin to meet people who are in the field of your bliss, and they open the doors to you. I say, follow your bliss and don't be afraid, and doors will open where you didn't know they were going to be."*
>
> *Joseph Campbell,* ***The Power of Myth***

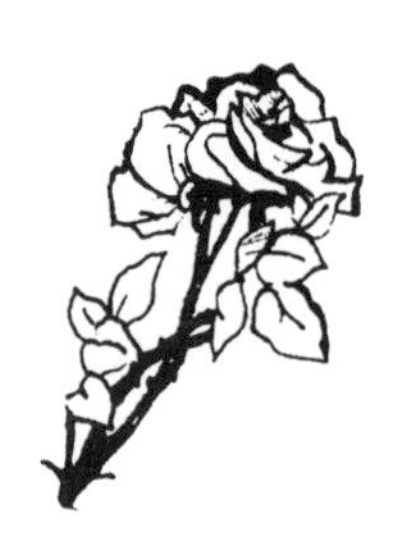

CHAPTER FORTY-THREE

IT WAS EASTER morning and my sense of isolation was deep. I had returned late the night before from five days of yet another inward bound cruise, this time as a back-up team member for a Cross Over seminar. Now I sat outside on my sunny patio steps, desultorily reviewing the week.

I didn't doubt that I had played a role in the movement of some of the people in the past week's seminar, and that there were those who learned some things from me. Yet there was a part of me that wanted confirmation and recognition of this. That was the part that doubted my gifts, that throughout the seminar had kept me on tenterhooks with its self-consciousness and pathetic desire for approval. I wondered, *How is it that the other team members and participants so effortlessly interacted with each other and with the trainers, Jerry and Kris? This issue of self-consciousness around powerful people is a huge wall for me. I want to transcend it.*

I had so desperately wanted to "make a good impression" that there was hardly a moment when I wasn't noticing and evaluating my performance. Only when I became totally involved with the participants did I get out of that self-conscious mode. *Being that way absolutely sucks. It's self-focusing, it separates me, it keeps me ineffective. It's also visible to anyone around me. As long as I don't get this issue handled, I'm going to be continually measuring and comparing myself with others.*

Picking up a brochure lying on my lap, I reread the description of Jerry's Vision Trek seminar, thinking, *This might be an arena where*

I can work through my self-consciousness issues. But the Vision Trek involved several days of backpacking in the desert. *Can my body do that?* I asked apprehensively. *I can find out*, I decided. Within half an hour, I had filled my daypack and was in my car headed for the Columbia Gorge and the Eagle Creek trail.

The Gorge was pristine and rugged. Heady waterfalls plummeted between rocky chasms and spring green was faintly emerging along the steep hillside meadows. How long it had been since I'd struck off on an adventure in this way. It seemed very necessary and important to be outside the city, outside my daily rounds and expectations.

As I hiked, I reviewed the Cross Over seminar. *Jerry and Kris must have found me icky sticky and sucky*, I thought. *Not in the sense of being all over them, but in the sense of my radiating neediness. My eyes must have looked like they were pleading for recognition. My body must have reflected my feelings of begging for acceptance from them. YUK!*

So Jerry and Kris both did the natural thing--turn away--refusing to support me in my game. It was the best thing for me, and it was the only attractive behavior for them. I felt totally discounted by them, felt that they considered me a lightweight, substanceless woman, and it was really about my own view of myself. It was ME, somehow, for some reason, saying that I was a lightweight person, *compared to certain others.*

The reasons why are not important, I realized. *The importance is in recognizing the behavior and changing it. This is truly a big issue for me. There is no way I'll ever be accepted in the world of powerful people until I accept myself as equally special and good enough. My life simply will not take off in the ways I want until I resolve this issue.*

Hence my desire to do Vision Trek and why I now stood on this high rocky point, the Columbia River yawning below like a great fiord. I had purposefully loaded the daypack to give weight. Although I feared finding out, I really wanted to know what my body could do. Trudging up and up the winding, tree-bordered trail, I had no problem. Granted, I took it easy and stopped often to sit and watch the river becoming a silver ribbon below me.

After three hours, I reached Wauna Point where a hip-high concrete obelisk stood alone in a clearing overlooking the distant river. *I did it. I have come this far in two and a half years.*

And what, indeed, **has** *brought me here?* I asked myself. *The diets? The exercise? The doctors, acupuncture, supplements and seminars and all the other therapies I've tried?* It was impossible to pinpoint one thing and say, "Ah-ha! That did it." *I think what really did it is what's happened in my head, in changing my attitude. Not just superficially, but deeply, at my core, changing my inner images, changing my self, and world, view.*

Leaning across the top of the obelisk, atop the mighty peak, amidst the comforting trees, the tears fell. What a long haul it had been back to myself, back to a place where my body reflected wholeness and could move again in nature. Gazing around me, I said, *I vow to use this gift, this energy and strength, daily. I vow to come into nature as often as I can to renew.*

> *"... Tune your ear*
> *To all the wordless music of the stars*
> *And to the voice of nature, and your heart*
> *Shall turn to truth and goodness as the plant*
> *Turns to the sun ..."*
>
> *Ralph Waldo Trine,* ***In Tune with the Infinite***

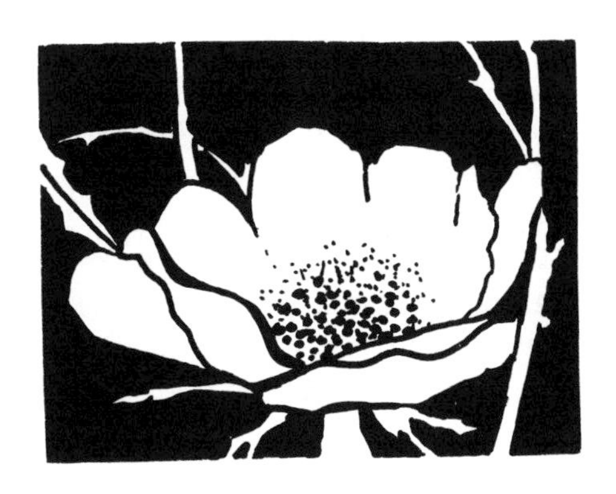

CHAPTER FORTY-FOUR

A COUPLE OF days after my climactic hike up to Wauna Point, I gave yet another friend a free massage. Once again, I was filled with delight, joy, and wonderment at the way things worked out without my doing a thing. I'd had such an urge toward giving Sally a massage, sensing that it would establish a connection from which other connections could develop. And that was just what happened. We visited all the while she was on the table. It wasn't until more than an hour and a half had passed and I began working on her head, that she started talking about her husband.

As she dressed, she continued talking--pouring out her concerns, fears and doubts about the manner in which they related. How I wished I had more skills. *Patience,* I told myself, *The skills are coming. At least the seminar trainings and my sessions with Steve are a start.* As Sally and I talked, I blessed my difficult experiences because everything (except the kids) that concerned Sally had happened to me in a similar way. The tight jaw and the mouth splint, the self-doubt and spinning out of control, the kind, but analytical and non-emotional husband.

*I **am** doing my "work." This is exactly what I want.* I loved the sense of being a source, a support, a dumping ground for people like Sally. I had the tapes and books and quotes to loan out for each situation. I'd experienced enough to be able to relate directly in almost all circumstances. *My experiences are my credentials, are they not?*

"The misery I have seen gives me strength, and faith in my fellow man supports my confidence in the future. I do hope I shall find a sufficient number of people who, because they themselves have been saved from physical suffering, will respond to those in need."

Albert Schweitzer, ***On the Edge of the Primeval Forest***

The next day was Saturday, and it was midnight before I sat down to write in my journal. Despite the late hour, energy pulsed through me after a rousing evening of songs with Carol and Trish. How I welcomed the renewal of such special events in my life. Only the week before I had reacquainted myself with nature, with moving through it actively. In the morning I had jogged for the longest stretches that I'd managed in three years ... and my legs felt great. And in the evening--Singing! I did not get tired. My voice was fluid and rich, my energy high. I could have easily continued past midnight.

It is a rebirthing of the events and activities of old, but different, I wrote in my journal. *I* ***involve*** *myself differently.* I was in the moment, immersed in the process, thoroughly involved in the enjoyment of the activity. If I wanted to try harmonizing, I did, without fears about doing it wrong. No holding back. No "trying" at all. I let the singing flow out naturally, trusting that whatever came out would be all right. I was thrilled by how good it sounded when I was in this mode of "taking no thought."

I remembered an incident from that morning, and thought, *Ah, James Newton, talented seminar trainer, how could you know what a gift, what a resource your words of recognition are*? My friend, Sharon, had phoned and told me what James said to the PES back-up team the previous week after I'd dropped off my contribution of their evening meal.

"That woman has it so well together. I just love being around her," and something about being a "many-talented woman." To think such words would come from such a man as James, a man whom I admired and respected and to whom I was attracted. What a measure of my metamorphosis in those difficult three years!

At the end of the week I flew once again to Santa Cruz. As I settled into my old bedroom with the picture windows looking out on a wild gully of oaks and cactus, I felt isolated and sad. I was thinking, *Here I am in the house that I've recognized as my family home for the last 15 years. It is the same. Yet the family is different.*

Sister, Dad and Mom had been at the airport waiting for me. What a motley group they made. Sis in her torn and dirty jeans straight from the horse barn. Dad stooped and looking wasted, in baggy green corduroy pants, a too-big grey sweater and his faded red stocking cap. Mom in her ancient red trousers and red sweater that she got at the Goodwill, her Goodwill blue coat over them, and her hair! Her hair was uncut, unpermed, nearly shoulder length, frizzy and grey, with bangs nearly to her eyebrows. She could easily have been taken for a bag lady. I thought, *All of them would be rounded up and taken to shelters if anyone found them roaming the streets.*

"Are you not getting your hair done anymore?" I had asked Mom.

"It's hard to get away. I don't like to leave Dad alone."

With Dad's illness, she had relinquished even more of her grip on reality. As if she inwardly threw up her hands and said, "I can't possibly cope." Who would ever discern the once well-coiffured community leader?

Who would perceive in Dad the once dapper lawyer and symphony musician, or in Mom the fastidious hostess reigning over the elegant house on the hill? They could afford anything they desired several times over, but had descended ever-deeper into their Depression-honed habits of thriftiness and clinging to what they had. It was also as if neither of them had the energy any more to keep up the front. *What does the appearance matter, after all?* I asked myself. I felt gentle and protective toward them. At the same time, I felt alien, as if I were from another orbit. And I seemed to have grown taller each time I came to Santa Cruz.

A couple of days later, I walked up to the wild, oak-studded park behind the house and met Dad at the Stroke Center. Back at home, we sat out on the sunny deck waiting for Mom and Sis to return with the house key. Without preliminaries Dad said, "I'll confide to you something I wouldn't tell anyone else."

My heart pounded. He'd never taken me into his personal confidences. Would I be able to respond appropriately?

"Yes?"

"At night when I lie awake I think about doing away with myself ... I wonder what's the point of continuing ... I feel like I screwed up by getting sick ... I can't get anything right ... I should have done better with Mom and Sis and organizing the taxes ..."

What do I say? I could only think, *Thank goodness, I'm sitting down.* My legs were quaking, my heart pounding faster. *Get the brain out of the way.*

"You did the best you could at the time."

His face cleared as he took in that idea. He was so unused to acknowledging his achievements.

"I admire and respect you very much for what you've done for me, for us all. It's meant so much to me how you've supported us and taken care of us." It seemed important to remind and reassure him that there *had* been successes. I didn't need to disclose the things I missed.

"You've provided safe, comfortable homes, wonderful trips and education ... You have no idea what your gift of the property money has meant to me this last year ..."

He brightened even more, "I'm glad to be told that."

I'd told him and Mom so many times, in letters or on the phone, but somehow it escaped him. Years before, when I was studying gymnastics in Denmark, I wrote them a heartful letter expressing my gratitude and awe at having been given such an experience. They never acknowledged it.

"I know you are concerned about the doctor bills. You know, I don't view the property money as 'mine,' I can always give some back if you ever need it."

I didn't protest his desire to "do away" with himself. Instead, I found myself saying, "I, too, know the feeling of hopelessness and pointlessness. I also know that 'this too shall pass.' You have a tremendous amount of healing to do from the stroke stuff and the brain surgery, and you're doing it. Once that levels off you will find that you can lead a very good life with the leukemia. People do--for years."

The words were flowing now, and I continued, "You know one characteristic I have is impatience ... and that is something you have too."

"Who me?" he asked with a sparkle in his eye.

"The process of healing is wonderful for learning the art of patience. Even now, as you simply sit in your chair, you are about the healing process. It takes time. Patience is necessary *and* is a by-product. St Augustine said, 'The reward of patience is patience.'"

Finally, having the courage to return to the initial subject, I said, "About your ending it, I enjoy having you around. I kind of like you."

"I guess I just don't have the courage to end it."

"Perhaps the courage is in staying."

That conversation with my father would become a touchstone for me ... a memory that I would look back on for the rest of my life. It was the crowning demonstration of the degree to which our relationship had evolved. We really *had* come closer to each other. It *wasn't* my imagination. I realized, too, that he desperately needed a confidant, a counselor of sorts. How sad it was to see both my parents arrive at such an age and state of their lives with no one they could call friend. They feared exposing and imposing themselves, and "wouldn't dream" of *asking* for anything. There was no one to whom they could express their true feelings. Once again, I was grateful for the lessons of my own illness, which had prepared me for this situation.

On the day of my departure, I drove away from Mom and Dad and Santa Cruz feeling discomforted about the leave-taking. In the final moments with them I had wanted to connect more deeply than to just talk at surface levels about "taking care" and "write some letters." I hugged them both and felt the awkwardness from Dad. He was heavily preoccupied with his day's "worries"--getting to the stroke center and then to the stock holders' meeting on time. He fussed and agonized about the most trivial details. But how could I pull him out of himself?

I felt sad about my family. They were so focused on being victims and on chanting their litany of woes: I don't have enough time; I don't have the right property; I don't have enough money; The government is screwed up; Medicare is a hassle; The auto mechanics are out to get us.

I so wished I had more counseling skills. The best I could do was to slow myself down and wait for the words to come. Repeatedly, I told myself, *This is where they are right now. I can do nothing except be close and try to recognize the truth, the wholeness, that is the true nature of their being.*

CHAPTER FORTY-FIVE

NO SOONER HAD I returned to Portland than I dived right back into my program of pushing myself to grow and change. I leaped at every chance to participate in situations where I could practice the opposite behavior to that which I'd always done. I embraced being in those circumstances which forced me to be focused in the moment and to respond and act out of a spontaneous, trusting, intuitive place. The opportunities were many and varied.

One Saturday in late April I helped Steve facilitate a firewalk workshop out at Diane's on the Sandy River. I found, to my surprise, that it was easy co-leading the trust falls, trust walks, and other preparatory processes throughout the day. As night fell, we lit the fire and my real work began: spraying down the grass, raking coals, pushing the fallen logs back onto the pile, spraying feet after people walked.

Everyone walked. Then we did a group walk. Steve picked me to lead it. We all walked a third time. I really wanted to break through my barriers, and I walked yet again. Afterwards, I realized with amazement that the whole event had been FUN. I'd had no fears, no body sensations at all. In the post-walk sharing, my delight bubbled over as I chattered, "What fun this has been! Who would have thought that a firewalk would be *fun*?!"

Driving home together in the star-studded midnight, Steve and I reviewed the day. "I can't believe how much fun it was," I burbled. "Just let me know if you ever need assistance again."

He asked, "Would your offer include a long weekend?"

I was momentarily confused. "A long firewalk? You mean one at the coast?"

"*Any* weekend seminar ... a Self-Acceptance, Transforming Fear, whatever."

I was blown away as I realized that Steve was talking about assisting in other seminars besides firewalks. He was offering me transformational work--what I'd been dreaming of.

A week later another new course was under way. I'd conducted my second allergy/candida cooking class in the big, modern facility of a local natural food store. Afterwards, even though I was dog-tired, I was too wound up to go to bed. Instead, I walked alone in the spring evening. The trees were ethereal in their showers of white blossoms, their new leaves brilliant under the street lights. I had such a sense of the presence of my mate. He was not physically there, yet I felt as if there was a presence walking with me.

I'd worked flat out all day preparing for the cooking class. In the morning, I'd been on the verge of cancelling it because there were only three people signed up. Then there were four, and I decided to go ahead. *After all,* I told myself, *the point is not what can I* ***get*** *out of this, what money can I earn? The point is that I am here to give.*

And that's what I asked throughout the day. *How may I serve these four people? What is it that they are coming to get from me?* I knew that I must step Barbara aside and let whatever it was flow out.

By evening two more people had joined the class, which I chose to approach differently than I had the last time. First, I got introductions from each person, along with their reason for being there. I shared my reasons for the class and then discussed the kinds of foods we would be using. I'd prepared most dishes ahead, and we started a half hour earlier, so it was comfortable and leisurely with plenty of time to eat, chat, answer questions, and exchange information.

At the end of the evening, one lady summed up her experience, saying, "What an informative and interesting class. I'm so glad I came." This was gratifying acknowledgment of the benefits of my letting it flow, especially as this comment came from the lady who'd been on the MS diet as well as the candida diet, and who'd already done a lot of learning about alternative food.

Even though the previous month's class had been horribly hectic and like a "mistake," I now found myself blessing it. For I had learned from it how I wanted to approach this night's class, and it worked so wonderfully well this new way.

> *"Praise yourself for your courage to make mistakes. Risking something new is the essence of learning."*
>
> *Read and Rusk, **I Want to Change, But I Don't Know How***

In early May, I once more put the rest of my life on hold and hopped aboard another Wings "cruise." The opportunity had come along for me to be a back-up team member for another Cross Over seminar, and I was ready to try my wings again. Once more, I found myself in an intense, eye-opening adventure. It was a week of being in the company of powerful, compassionate, integrous people. A week of watching the transformation of committed, seeking people. I received feedback that validated my own sense of having moved and changed. My body was, for the most part, strong. Despite the late hours and early rising, I slept well. People asked me about myself and wanted to know what I did.

The ultimate measure of my progress came on the last night. Bev, the trainer, who knew me only from the previous August's Cross Over, told me, "You were so real." (up in front of the group) "You were in your element, and you were clear and real. People get that and they respond."

The trainings always moved me--always taught me so much. This one represented a recognition of my solidness, of my gifts, of moving away from self-doubt to the awareness of myself as a resource for the participants.

At home I picked a Rune for this last Cross Over: BREAKTHROUGH.

A few days later, more new experiences of growth took place. I drove to the coast with Steve for my first long weekend of assisting him in a workshop. In typical Steve fashion, he offered me few clues as to what I could expect. I was nervous, but eager to see how I'd do in these new circumstances.

In the early afternoon, Steve, Susan and I settled into our rooms at the old hotel high on a cliff over the Pacific Ocean. The seminar participants would not come for another two hours. Within ten minutes of arriving, Steve unpacked several foot-long pine boards.

Balancing one of these between the backs of two chairs, he karate chopped it with his hand. Then turning to me and Susan, he said, "Your turn."

The offer came up so unexpectedly and so fast that I didn't have time to collect my beliefs and my inabilities or my fears about getting hurt. Steve demonstrated how to hold my hand sideways to the wood, how to raise it up and come down hard. He said, "It's just like a firewalk. You commit to breaking it. You hit it hard and you just know when you are ready."

Susan had declined, so I went first. I simply did it. Steve had done it and I trusted his guidance completely. The board snapped in two. Simple. My hand stung for a couple of moments and then NOTHING. No residue, no pain, no bruise. Not even an "Ah ha!" in my brain. It just seemed like the most logical, natural thing to have done.

> *"Belief systems are only belief systems and not realities ... Once we realize that we live only in an idea level of existence that is not based on any intrinsic realness, we may consider the possibility that* ***there are options to our experience and expression of reality****."*
>
> *Brugh Joy,* ***Joy's Way***

I was delighted to discover that I easily related to the weekend group, easing myself into the role of assistant. I made a good liaison between the several women and Steve and Susan, Steve's other assistant. Not that the group wasn't connected. It was just a nice dimension to have a sort of middle person. I discovered that I could both participate *and* lead. I supported and led from within the group. It was clear what *I* was there for--to learn about trust and leadership.

On the second day of the retreat, I was given the chance to really stretch myself. For "Soap Opera Theater," Steve asked me to perform a monologue of *my* Soap Opera. What to do? I'd left so much stuff behind. I felt that I'd grown beyond soap operas. Gradually, though, inspiration flickered. For this group of women who saw themselves as "done-to" by men, I offered a monologue on how to keep a man distant: Never be honest; Never tell him what's on your mind; Always avoid touchy or emotional issues; Don't be vulnerable; Don't tell him privately what's bothering you. Instead, save it up for some public opportunity where you can bait him or embarrass him with snide, underhanded remarks; Never ask for what you want, and always expect him to be a mind reader ...

Good or bad? It didn't matter. The women laughed, and I believed that they got the message about how we play these games which keep men, and women, distant from us.

At the end of the retreat, we shared the significance of the Angel cards we each picked. I had drawn FREEDOM. It seemed appropriate. Yes, a reflection of the changed me. I'd let go of, and was free of, the old behaviors with men and sex and self-consciousness. Weekends like this and the PES and Cross Over back-up teams validated for me the measure of my freedom from the old constraints and concepts. I felt freer than ever to follow my heart and to trust at levels I never had before.

> *"The true value of a human being is judged only by the extent that he is freed of himself."*
>
> *Einstein*

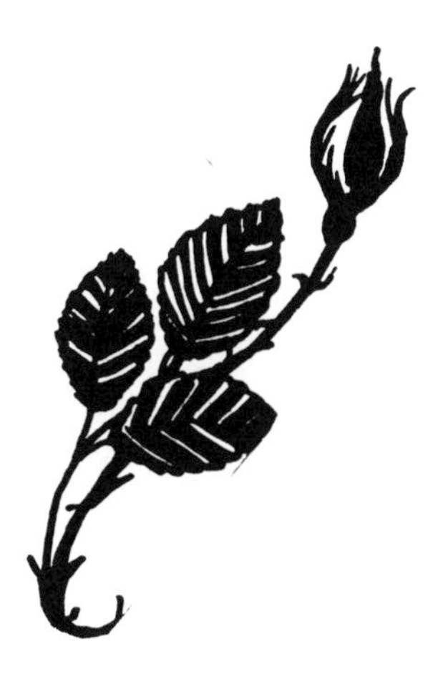

CHAPTER FORTY-SIX

IT WAS NEARLY the end of May, and I was spending the weekend at Diane's on the Sandy River. The first night was spent soaking luxuriously in the hot tub with Diane and another friend, Beverly. We three lounged in the hot water on the high deck looking straight out at the tops of the maples and firs rising from the river which hummed merrily below us. How grand and warm was the contrast of the hot, silky water with the dark, whispering leaves and the chill breeze all around. I reflected, *In other years I would have felt guilty about my good fortune and would have questioned how I should be so deserving of such good friends and of such pleasure. Tonight, I accept it.*

I gazed with Beverly and Diane at the distant clouds swiftly drifting across the sky. We could see the white glow where the moon must be hidden. As we watched, the line of running clouds narrowed and dipped until, at last, their peaks dropped below the level of the moon. Suddenly the full moon shone forth in all its white glory, only to be darkened once again by yet another squadron of flitting clouds. They raced passed and soon the moon burst forth again. Just like the shadow-play of my life.

The next day, Diane, Beverly and I had a high, rollicking time together. We started with hot tubbing and then eating fruit and pancakes as we sprawled across the floor of the log-walled living room where a fire danced in the stone fireplace.

The day was grey and showery, but indoors it was so warm that I was happy to dress in T-shirt and panties. Diane was eager to show us her special swimming hole, so after breakfast we hiked down to the river and along its bank, Diane's two big dogs romping ahead of us. This was all private property and I had such a sense of peace and security. After half a mile, we reached the area, absolutely pristine, where the river was wide and smooth and, despite its name, clear. The white beach was clean and spacious. A rocky cliff rose on the bank immediately ahead of us, effectively cutting off land access from upriver.

I was enchanted by the spirit of the place, and felt warmed and touched by Diane's enthusiasm. She unabashedly loved her property and these special spots, and loved sharing them with her friends. Her delight and enjoyment were so appealing, so catching.

Soon my life would be bound up in this magical place and this river. How could I then imagine the connection I would one day have with this spot, in sun and rain, and tears and laughter, or that one day it would be my wedding site?

Later that afternoon, Diane and Beverly drove me back to town. As they deposited me at home, we were teasing each other about meeting men. Both girls started talking about Sid.

"Who is Sid?" I asked.

They exchanged looks and squealed, and Beverly said, "Sid is *perfect* for Barbara!"

They'd mentioned Sid throughout the weekend: "Sid installed the electric gate. Sid fixed the lawn tractor. Sid built the deck. Sid installed the hot tub. Sid takes me kyacking." I'd paid no attention.

Now Diane told me more about Sid, "Sid is a retired electrician. He lives across the river. He's my handyman. He loves to do things for other people."

"Is he single?"

"No, he's married, but he and his wife lead separate lives. They're getting a divorce. I think he's really lonely."

"Why would he be so perfect for me?"

"He's always interested in meeting interesting people. He's a heart person. He's really open. He's even done a firewalk. He was here for the walk that Channel 10 filmed. He's a neat guy."

I was intrigued with the idea of being considered as a possibility for a meeting with *any* man. I was careful to put no expectations on such things, but admittedly enjoyed the heightened sense of anticipation that came with the proposed meeting. Part of me longed for companionship, but I wondered, *Do I want that sort of elemental disruption?* I assured myself, *Never mind. It's most unlikely that anything will come of it. Let it be. WHATEVER.*

Thus was set in motion the final step bringing me to my destiny. An introductory dinner was planned for Diane's big farm kitchen. Beverly was present as a safe, neutral party. At six o'clock, a tall, wiry man with iron-gray curly hair strolled in and presented each of us ladies with a rose wrapped in green paper. He was wearing jeans and a plaid wool shirt and struck me as looking uncomfortably rigid. In my first impression I judged, *No, this isn't the one.* I noted his lean build and thought, *How could I possibly be in a relationship with a man whose thighs are thinner than mine*?

After a carefully polite dinner, Diane and Beverly discreetly disappeared while Sid and I remained lounging on the living room floor in the dancing light of the wood fire. Unexpectedly, I found that the conversation easily ebbed and flowed. This was the first inkling I had of the surprises that were in store for me from this man.

In fact, Sid was perfect for me, like an angel dispensed from heaven who knew my needs better than I did. Sid was, indeed, the man who would satisfy that longing for nurturing, companionship, and love that had been building within me.

Meeting Sid would *not* resolve the issues of my life. In some ways it would create more. I had grown accustomed to my privacy and solitude and personal growth pursuits. I would have to learn how to balance that with the requirements of a partner. I was still growing and changing at deep and varied levels. I would have to learn to accommodate another's needs despite whatever confusions might stir me. My body, with its pattern of plateaus and backsliding, would continue pressing me for restrictions, treatments, or rest when my only desire was to be active and participating with Sid and with life.

Yet Sid's presence would change the entire character of my quest for health and wholeness. I was no longer alone. In the times ahead Sid would be the person I could complain to or cry with. No longer would I have to make decisions from my solitary judgment. He would step into worlds completely beyond his past experience as he opened to the many and strange ways he could support me in the struggle.

He learned massage so that he could offer relief to my aching buttocks and legs. He learned to give lymph drains and how to assist in my cooking classes. He watched doctors pounding or pricking my body and cried with me. He came swimming with me and ate vegetables for breakfast, lunch and dinner. When we walked together, he slowed his steps to accommodate mine or lifted me off my feet to give me rest. He became friends with my friends.

Eventually, Sid gave me the ultimate gift of my writing, because he entered the world of computers in order to teach it to me. At every level, he offered me love, friendship, nurturing, support, and recognition such as I'd never dreamed could exist.

And the nature of my growth began to change. Gradually, the pattern of growth through suffering gave way to the recognition that I was growing and changing and releasing through JOY. With it, the body increasingly reflected greater degrees of wellness. Unbelievably, my health and my life began to take on the qualities that I had dreamed of, but doubted could happen.

As John Honse had predicted, my life was indeed turned on its head. As I continued my inner and outer stretching, the increased wholeness of my life was reflected not only in a well body, but also in an incredible and unimagined abundance of experiences, people, and travel. Within that first year, Sid and I spent a month exploring the San Juan Islands on his little boat, visited Vancouver's Expo, celebrated Thanksgiving with my family in California, trekked like children to Disneyland and then to Mexico, and rafted down Oregon's Rogue River.

And that was only the beginning. The story unfolds in ever increasing circles of joy--joy and trust, opening and growing, and releasing ever further the beliefs that tell us we cannot live in freedom, abundance, happiness, purpose. It is another story, and one that I shall eventually share; how with continued commitment to shedding our beliefs in limitation, and to jointly honoring and opening to ALL that is possible, the unfoldment of our lives has taken on the character almost of a fairytale.

Dreams do come true. I write the final pages of this book in Australia, the land to which I always dreamed of returning, and where my writing has taken on a new flavor. I write of adventure and exploration and joy in each moment, of camel rides on pristine beaches and swimming in moonlit tropical pools, of rugged mountain climbs and desert treks, of rich reunion with old friends and of meeting and counseling new ones.

For as Sid and I opened, the world opened to us--across the United States and across the world. I see this opening as a reflection of the increased wholeness within myself, a wholeness which today shows up in a strong, healthy body that, for the most part, runs, plays squash and racquetball, and eats "normally." It is a wholeness that derives from a continued commitment to seeking the truth about who and what I am. It requires that I continually give forth the lessons of the last several years, in each moment, with each person, in each place, never doubting that ANYTHING IS POSSIBLE.

> *"Would you be willing*
> *to get out of your own way,*
> *and let the miracles that are yours*
> *by divine right come into your life?"*
> *Rusty Berkus,* ***Appearances***

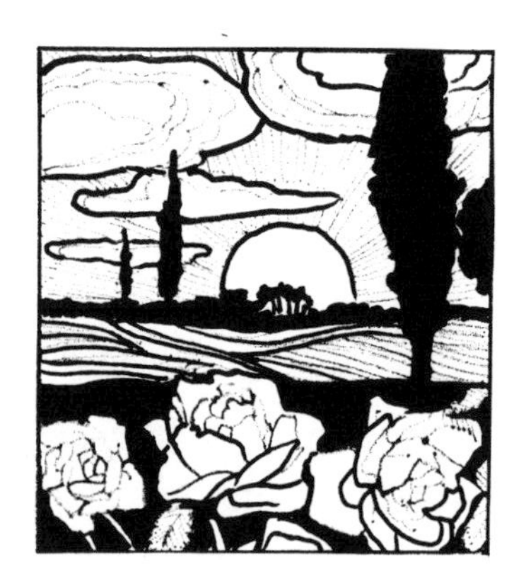

Not the End, but a New Beginning

READING LIST

Acterberg, Jean Ph.D. *Imagery in Healing*. Boston. Shambhala:1985.

Anonymous. *The Impersonal Life*. Marina del Rey. DeVorss: 1983.

Anonymous. *The Way Out*. Marina del Rey, DeVorss: 1971.

Allan, John. *The Healing Energy of Love; A Personal Journal*. Wheaton, Il. Theosophical Publishing House: 1986.

Bach, Richard. *Illusions*. New York. Dell: 1977.

Backhouse, Halcyon, Ed. *The Cloud of Unknowning*. London. Hodder & Stoughton: 1985.

Bartlet, John. *Familiar Quotations*. n.p. Little, Brown and Co.

Berkus, Rusty. *Appearances*. Encino, Ca. Red Rose Press: 1986.

Blum, Ralph. *The Book of Runes*. New York. St. Martin's Press: 1982.

Boone, J. Allen. *Kinship with All Life*. New York. Harper & Row: 1976.

Brilliant, Ashley. *I Feel Much Better, Now That I've Given Up Hope*. Santa Barbara, CA. Woodbridge Press: 1984.

---. *I Have Abandoned My Search for Truth, and Am Looking for a Good Fantasy*. Santa Barbara, CA. Woodbridge Press: 1980.

---. *All I Want Is a Warm Bed and a Kind Word and Unlimited Power*. Santa Barbara, CA. Woodbridge Press: 1986.

Brother Lawrence. *The Practice of the Presence of God*. Garden City, New York. Image Books: 1977.

Buscaglia, Leo, Ph.D. *Living, Loving and Learning*. New York. Fawcett Columbine, 1982.

Buscaglia, Leo, Ph.D. *Personhood*. Thorofare, N.J., C.B.Slack: 1978.

Caddy, Eileen. *Word to Live By*. (Audio tape) Findhorn Press, 1971.

Campbell, Joseph with Bill Moyers. *The Power of Myth*. New York. Doubleday: 1988 (also on video).

Claremont de Castillejo, Irene. *Knowing Woman*. New York. Putnam: 1973.

Coffey-Lewis, Lou. *Be Restored to Health*. New York. Ballantine Books/Epiphany Edition: 1984.

Crook, William G., M.D. *The Yeast Connection*. Jackson, Tennessee. Professional Books: 1983.

Dass, Ram. *Journey of Awakening*. New York. Bantam: 1978.

Daumal, Rene. *Mount Analogue*. Baltimore. Penguin: 1952.

Diamond, Carlin. *Love It, Don't Label It!* San Rafael. Fifth Wave Press, 1985.

Emerson, Ralph Waldo. *Selected Essays, Lectures and Poems*. New York. Pocket Books: 1975.

Ferguson, Marilyn. *The Aquarian Conspiracy*. Los Angeles. Tarcher: 1980.

Foster, Richard J. *Celebration of Discipline*. New York. Harper & Row: 1988.

Gawler, Ian. *You Can Conquer Cancer*. Melbourne, Hill of Content: 1984.

Golas, Thaddeus. *The Lazy Man's Guide to Enlightenment*. New York. Bantam: 1981.

Goldsmith, Joel. *The Infinite Way*. (Plus many other books) Marina del Rey. DeVorss: 1984.

Gordon, Arthur. *A Touch of Wonder*. New York. Jove Books: 1974.

Hammarskjold, Dag. *Markings*. London. Faber: 1964.

Hazelden Meditation Series. *Each Day a New Beginning*. Minneapolis. Winston/ Hazelden: 1982.

Horn, Frances. *I Want One Thing*. Marina del Rey, CA. DeVorss & Co: 1981.

Illich, Ivan. *Medical Nemesis*. New York, Bantam, 1979.

Jampolsky, Jerry. *Love Is Letting Go of Fear*. Milbrae, CA. Celestial Arts: 1979.

Joy, W. Brugh, M.D.. *Joy's Way*. Los Angeles. Tarcher: 1979.

Keyes Jr., Ken. *Handbook to Higher Consciousness*. St. Mary, KY, Living Love Publications: 1975.

Kopp, Sheldon. *If You Meet the Buddha on the Road, Kill Him*. Ben Lomond, CA. Science & Behavior Books: 1972.

Kubler-Ross, M.D., Elisabeth. *On Death and Dying*. New York, Macmillan, 1969.

Leshan, Lawrence. *How to Meditate*. New York. Bantam. 1975.

Levine, Stephen. *A Gradual Awakening*. Anchor Books: 1979.

---.(Video) *Conscious Living: Conscious Dying*. n.p.

---. *Who Dies?* Garden City, N.Y. Anchor Press/Doubleday: 1982.

Levine, Stephen and Ram Dass. (Video) *The Heart of the Healer*. n.p.

MacLaine, Shirley. *It's All In The Playing*. Bantam: 1988.

---. *Out On A Limb*. Bantam: 1985.

Mandell, M. *Dr. Mandell's 5-Day Allergy Relief System*. New York, Pocket Books, 1979.

Mandini, Og. *The Greatest Salesman in the World.* New York. Bantam: 1968.

Mascaro, Juan, translator. *The Bhagavad Gita.* Penquin: 1962.

May, Rollo. *The Courage to Create.* New York. Bantam: 1975.

Merton, Thomas. *New Seeds of Contemplation.* New York. New Directions Books: 1962.

Millman, Dan. *The Way of the Peaceful Warrior.* Tiburon. H.J. Kramer, Inc.: 1980.

Oyle, Irving, M.D. *The New American Medicine Show.* Santa Cruz, CA. Unity Press: 1979.

Paton, Alan. *Instrument of Thy Peace.* New York. Ballantine/ Epiphany: 1968.

Ponder, Catherine. *The Dynamic Laws of Healing.* Marina del Rey, CA. DeVorss: 1985.

Powell, John. *Unconditional Love.* Valencia, CA. Tabor: 1978.

Ravindra, Ravi. *Whispers from the Other Shore.* Wheaton, IL. Theosophical Publishing House: 1984.

Rusk, Tom, M.D., and Read, Randy, M.D. *I Want to Change, But I Don't Know How!* Los Angeles. Price Stern Sloan: 1978.

Siegel, Bernie, M.D. *Love, Medicine, and Miracles.* Boston. G.K. Hall: 1986.

Simonton, Carl and Mathews-Simonton, Stephanie. *Getting Well Again.* New York. Bantam: 1978.

Sinetar, Marsha. *Do What You Love, The Money Will Follow.* New York. Paulist Press: 1987.

Vaughn, Frances, Ph.D. and Walsh, Roger, Ph.D. *Accept This Gift.* Los Angeles. Tarcher: 1983.

---. *The Gift of Peace.* Los Angeles. Tarcher: 1986.

Westbeau, Georges H. *Little Tyke.* Wheaton, Il. Theosophical Publishing House: 1986.

Winokur, Jon, Ed. *Zen To Go.* New York. New American Library: 1989.

Yogananda, Paramahansa. *The Law of Success.* The Self-Realization Fellowship, CA: 1974.

BOOKS BY OR ABOUT SURVIVORS

Bickel, Lennard. *Mawson's Will.* New York. Stein & Day: 1977.

Burgess, Perry. *Who Walk Alone.* New York. H. Holt & Co: 1940.

Callahan, Steven. *Adrift.* New York. Ballantine: 1986.

Cousins, Norman: *Anatomy of an Illness.* New York. W.W. Norton and Co: 1979.

Davidson, Robyn. *Tracks.* New York. Pantheon: 1980.

Eareckson, Joni. *Joni.* Grand Rapids, Michigan. Zondervan Corp: 1976.

Frank, Anne. *The Diary of a Young Girl.* n.p.

Franklin, Miles. *My Brilliant Career.* New York. St. Martin's Press: 1980.

---. *The End of My Career.* New York. St. Martin's Press: 1981.

Gann, Ernest. *Hostage to Fortune.* New York. Knopf: 1978.

Humard, Hannah. *Thou Shalt Remember: Lessons of a Lifetime.* New York. Harper & Row: 1988.

Kanin, Garson. *Kate* (biography of Katherine Hepburn) n.p.

Keneally, Thomas. *Schindler's List.* New York. Penguin: 1982.

Gill, Derek. *Quest: The Life of Elisabeth Kubler-Ross.* New York. Ballantine: 1982.

Ireland, Jill. *Life Wish.* New York. Jove Books: 1987.

Lovell, Mary S. *Straight on til Morning.* (The biography of Beryl Markham) New York. St. Martin's Press: 1988.

Markham, Beryl. *West With the Night.* San Francisco. North Point Press: 1983.

Moorehead, Alan. *Coopers Creek.* Great Britain. Hamilton. 1963.

Murphy, Dervla. *Where the Indus is Young; Walking to Baltistan.* London. Arrow: 1977.

---. *Wheels Within Wheels.* New Haven. Ticknor & Fields: 1980.

O'Hara, Mary. *The Scent of Roses.* London. M. Joseph: 1980.

Radner, Gilda. *It's Always Something.* New York. Simon & Schuster; 1989.

Read, Piers Paul. *Alive.* New York. Avon: 1974.

Sarton, May. *The Bridge of Years.* New York. W.W.Norton: 1985.

---. *Journal of a Solitude.* New York. W.W.Norton: 1973.

Smith, David. *Healing Journey, An Uncommon Athelete.* San Francisco. Sierra Club Books: 1983.

Stevenson, William. *A Man Called Intrepid.* New York. Ballantine: 1976.

Sullivan, Tom. *If You Could See What I Hear.* New York. Signet: 1976.

Thomas, Lowell. *Good Evening, Everybody.* New York. Morrow: 1976.

Thompson, Thomas: *Lost!* New York. Atheneum: 1975.

Wax, Judith. *Starting in the Middle.* New York. Fawcett: 1979.

West, Jessamyn. *The Woman Said Yes.* Har. Brace J: 1986.

---. *To See the Dream.* London. Hodder & Stoughton: 1958.

Wilby, Sorrel. *Tibet; A Woman's Lone Trek Across A Mysterious Land,* Melbourne. MacMillan Co: 1988.

Weedon, Dianne. *Tears in My Champagne.* Brisbane. Champagne Publications: 1984.

AVAILABLE FROM FOUR WINDS PUBLICATIONS

JOURNEY TO WHOLENESS; *And the day came when the risk to remain tight in a bud was more painful than the risk it took to bloom*, by Barbara Marie Brewster. $14.95 U.S. $19.95 Aus.

DOWN UNDER ALL OVER; *A Love Affair With Australia* by Barbara Marie Brewster. $14.95 U.S. $19.95 Aus.

DOWN UNDER ALL OVER photocards by Barbara Brewster. Moments and places in Australia as depicted in the book ***Down Under All Over***. 6" x 4" mounted glossy color prints. Packaged in poly sleeve. $2.50 each US. For a list of card subjects send request to Four Winds Publishing.

SHIPPING: In the U.S., including Alaska and Hawaii, add $3 for the first book and $1 for each additional title shipped to the same address. Books are shipped UPS or first class mail. Canadian orders, please add $4 U.S. for the first book and $2 U.S. for each additional title sent to the same address.

A GIFT? Just supply us with the name and address. Orders promptly shipped. Prices are subject to change without notice.

FOUR WINDS PUBLISHING:
6267 S.W. Miles Ct.
Portland, Oregon, 97219, USA.
Phone: (503) 246-9424 FAX: (503) 246-9497

IN AUSTRALIA DIRECT REQUESTS TO:
FOUR WINDS PUBLISHING
Box 752, Naracoorte
South Australia, 5271.
Phone: 087-62-0113 FAX: 087-62-0104